MAD DOGS AND ENGLISHMEN WENT OUT IN THE QUEENSLAND SUN

Health aspects of the settlement of tropical Queensland

THE BANCROFT ORATION OF 1969

by

Douglas Gordon

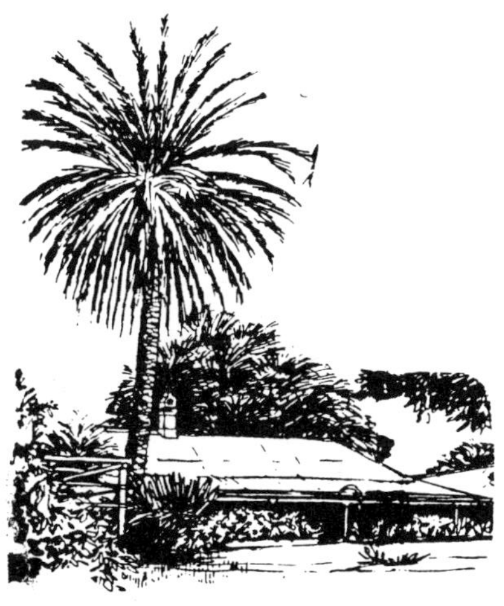

Amphion Press
1990

MAD DOGS AND ENGLISHMEN WENT OUT IN THE QUEENSLAND SUN

Bibliography
Illustrations
Notes and References
Includes Index

1st Edition (English)
First Published 1990

Author: Emeritus Professor Douglas Gordon

Typeset and Published by: Amphion Press
(Department of Child Health Publishing Unit)
Department of Child Health, University of Queensland,
Royal Children's Hospital, Brisbane, Q. 4029. Australia.

Printed by: The University Printery, The University of Queensland,
St Lucia, Brisbane, Q. 4067. Australia.

Cover by: Paul Ramsden and Robert Allen, The Queensland Museum.

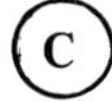 Douglas Gordon

CATALOGUING IN PUBLICATION DATA
National Library of Australia
Gordon, Douglas (1911-   )

Mad Dogs and Englishmen went out in the Queensland Sun

1. Tropical Medicine — Queensland — History.
2. Pioneers — Health and hygiene — Queensland — History.
3. Queensland — Industries — History. I. Title
614.42943
NATIONAL LIBRARY OF AUSTRALIA CARD NUMBER AND ISBN
ISBN 0 86776 359 0

CONTENTS

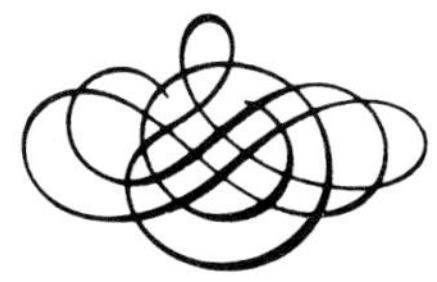

The subject of heat is one of extreme delicacy in Queensland,

as indeed, it is also in the other colonies.

One does not allude to heat in a host's house,

any more than to a bad bottle of wine

or an ill-cooked joint of meat.[1]

It is so hot that people going from it to an evil place

are said to send back to earth for their blankets,

finding that evil place to be too chilly for them

after the home they have left.[1] *

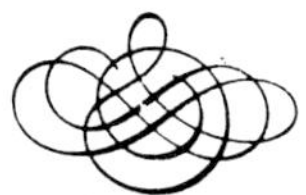

**This quotation from Trollope referred to his visit to
Rockhampton which took place in winter time.*

PREFACE

Advances in the quality of life and in better health, and in the prevention of disease come about because of men's and women's adaptation to new environments, and to the adoption of new knowledge. Such also result from a society's will to invest in such unspectacular resources as good drainage, good sanitation, rigid control on the quality and supply of food and water, and on the development of suitable housing.

The settlement of northern Australia saw the evolution of all these themes in an environment deemed hostile, not by its indigenous inhabitants from the preceding twenty millennia, but by the latter day caucasian and oriental pioneers who partly supplanted them. The lessons of this latter adaptation are important ones for societies of the future. It is fitting that one learns of some of these, in this account.

The Bancroft Oration was established by the Queensland Branch of the British Medical Association in 1926 to honour its most respected scientist, Joseph Bancroft. This monograph sets out in some detail the Oration given by Douglas Gordon in 1969. In it he trenchantly develops the thesis that North Queensland was successfully settled from the 1860s onwards, mainly because of three industries and the calibre of the men and women in them. These were: pastoral activity, mining and sugar cane farming. There was a minor input from timber getting. These industries followed one after the other and were mutually supportive. They made the North Queensland area financially viable.

It so happens that Professor Gordon was uniquely fitted to discuss the relationship between industry and health in Queensland. He was brought up on a small grazing property at Tiaro on the northern foothills of Mt Bauple [Bopple]. This place is of significance in local Queensland history because it was there that the Aborigines of the Wide Bay district periodically enjoyed the Macadamia nuts which grew on the mountain.

At that place and time, boarding schools were necessary for the extended education of the country's youth. After a short period of primary schooling in Queensland, Douglas Gordon attended High School in New South Wales, and the first year of the medical course at Melbourne University in 1930. In the financially depressed years of the 1930s he worked first as a stockman and timber getter and later developed a dairy and sugar farm with a small contract ploughing business. When financial affairs improved he went back to medical school.

Douglas Gordon graduated in medicine from the University of Queensland in 1942 and in due course became a medical officer in the RAAF. While overseas in what is now Indonesia he was a medical officer to Airfield Construction squadrons. The other officers were engineers of various kinds. He became fascinated with the very practical knowledge these men had about accidents and sickness in industry.

So much was this so that, when the State Health Department in Queensland advertised for a medical officer to take charge of industrial hygiene [later termed industrial medicine], Douglas Gordon applied for the position and was accepted. He worked in this capacity between 1946 and 1957. During this period he studied the adaptation of workers to hot environments, carried out accident surveys, and could claim to have visited almost every mine and pit in the state. He was particularly involved in problems at Mt Isa, where the deep workings caused extremely hot conditions underground.

He visited North Queensland regularly and became entranced by the mystery of those coastal fevers which were still undiagnosed.

In 1957 the University of Queensland appointed Douglas Gordon as the first Professor of Preventive & Social Medicine in Australia, and he was the last of the Faculty of Medicine's part-time Deans (1963–67). He retired in 1976.

By the 1960s formal medical teaching had belatedly acknowledged the way in which the physical environment and socio-economic conditions affected health. The North Queensland area was particularly severe on human skin. When people are unemployed in our kind of society, they are usually poor. Nutrition, housing and personal cleanliness often suffer where there is poverty. Dr [later Sir] Raphael Cilento years before had described how meanly some people lived in North Queensland. Douglas Gordon claims that the remedies which were applied in the early decades of this century were successful because financially viable industries could pay for them. A nomadic indigenous population and the availability of reasonable communications also helped.

In this account, someone with a wide perspective presents an interpretation of the evolution of good health in northern Australia. Thus from the studied and interpreted past come the guidelines for tomorrow.

Professor John Pearn
Deputy Dean
The Faculty of Medicine
University of Queensland.

January 1990

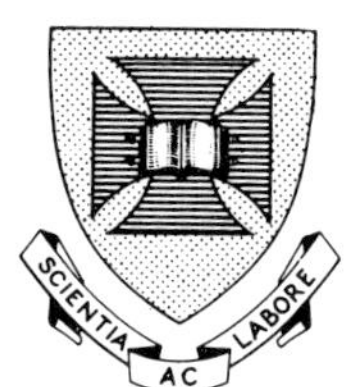

INTRODUCTION

In the 1860s North Queensland and western Queensland were settled by venturesome pastoralists who were drawn ever onwards by the prevailing "land hunger"of nineteenth century Australia. (*Fig. 1*) And thus members of a northern European people, without thinking very much about it, became permanent tropical dwellers. They became the only group of northern Europeans to successfully make a tropical lowlands their home. (Later there were Germans in Brazil.) White children were born there, educated there and lived out their entire lives in the hot parts of the new colony.

These northerners certainly did not seem to worry unduly about possible adverse effects to their health. In fact, the Registrar-General[2] in 1865 attested to the salubrious nature of the climate at Cape York, and in this he was supported by Dr Haran[3] the naval medical officer at Somerset where the Port of Refuge for Torres Strait was situated. Later, in 1884, Dr Jee[4] a medical practitioner who knew the Gulf country and the Peninsula quite well, was to say much the same thing. For several decades after North Queensland was first settled optimism about health seemed to be the usual attitude.[5]

These foolhardy settlers, however, obviously had not read the scientific text books which in those days took a gloomy view about white settlement in the tropics. Inevitable ill health and "racial degeneracy" were considered to be the principal limiting factors to permanent living in a tropical climate. The valiant empire builders always had taken regular "long leaves" from their arduous and dangerous responsibilities in the hotter climates. And finally colonial service usually was rewarded with early retirement to the recuperative environment of "home".

For reasons which we will discuss later, this North Queensland experiment became the subject of mordant controversy around the turn of the century. Since the effect of hot climates on health and on continuing human efficiency was at the centre of this debate, Australian doctors were deeply, and often emotionally, involved. The clinical and scientific arguments continued on down to World War II.

But in that War large numbers of soldiers from temperate climates lived and fought in the tropics without massive outbreaks of sickness. And since then we have committed huge sums of money to mineral and agricultural development in Northern Australia. Though the economics of the farming ventures have attracted much adverse criticism[6] the ability of the work force to remain healthy and to withstand climate stress is now taken for granted. It is considered pointless to worry unduly about ill health due to the climate in Northern Australia, provided that suitable housing, diet and attractive amenities are readily available.

The dust of contention has thus settled; and the sound and the fury have departed from arguments which once were bitter. It is therefore a fitting time to discuss why north Europeans were able to settle in tropical Queensland without any great amount of ill health relative to the prevailing disease patterns of those times.

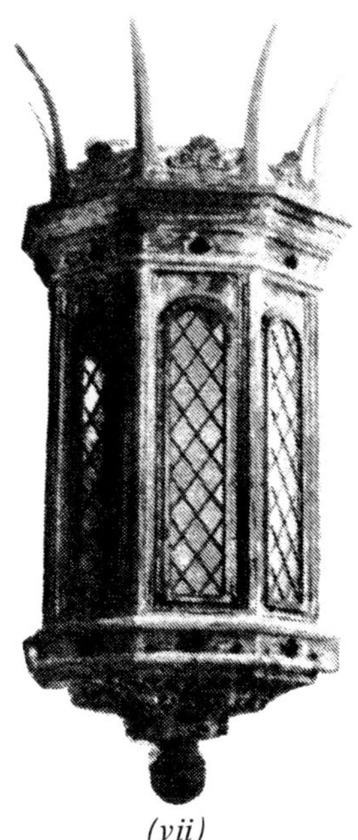

ACKNOWLEDGEMENTS ......

When I prepared the material for this Oration more than twenty years ago I received help from a number of libraries on the eastern coast of Australia and from numerous people. The text gives an indication of the extent of this assistance. Unfortunately, the changes which occur with retirement have erased the details of these sources.

Of greater relevance is the help which I have received in the present. The publication of this monograph would not have been possible without the expert knowledge and practical enthusiasm of Professor John Pearn and his editorial assistant Mrs Peggy Carter. I am indebted to Mr Paul Ramsden and to Mr Robert Allen for the cover graphics and art work.

I also have benefited greatly by reading the 1977 paper by Dr R.A. Douglas (*see p. 79*). As always my wife Joan has provided much clerical assistance.

Illustrations, unless stated otherwise, first appeared in the Annual Reports of the Commissioner of Public Health, for the State of Queensland, in approximately the first two decades of this century.

Douglas Gordon
Jindalee, Brisbane

1990

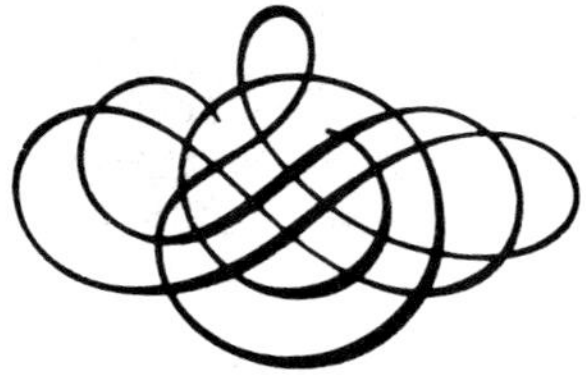

PART I

THE PHYSICAL ENVIRONMENT

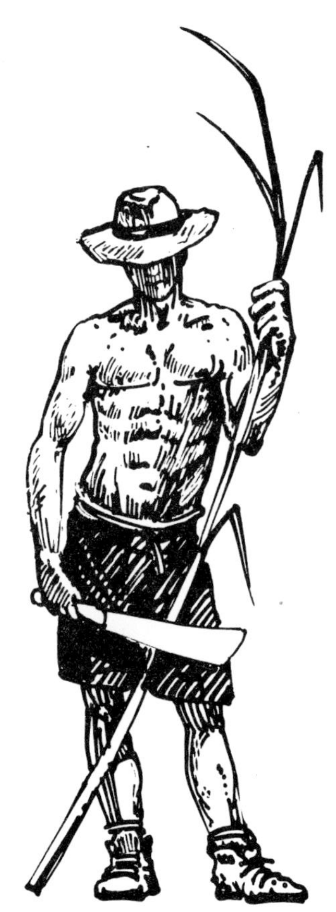

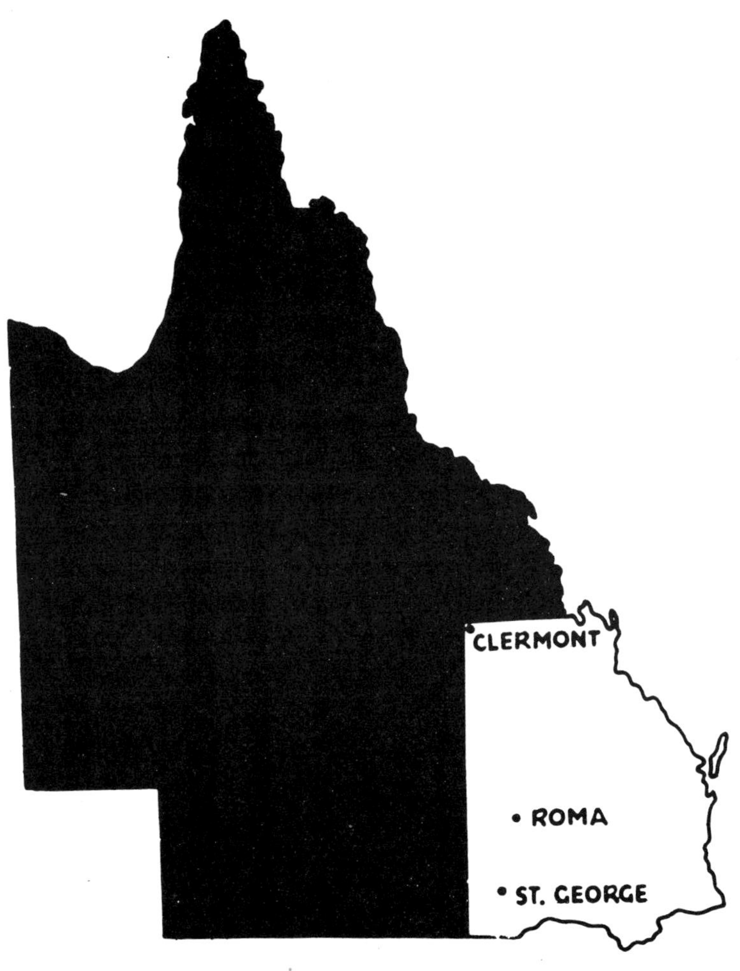

QUEENSLAND
AREA OF SETTLEMENT AT SEPARATION.

Figure 1: Most of the area appearing as 'black' on the map was settled during the 1860s.

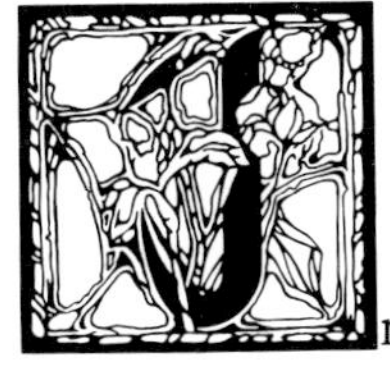n this part I will discuss:

- The firmly held belief that tropical residence was dangerous for white men.

- The nature of the North Queensland climate.

- The thesis which I will develop in this paper.

THE ALLEGED DANGERS OF TROPICAL RESIDENCE

The conviction that tropical climates were lethal to members of the white race found formal expression in the doctrine of "climatic determinism". As quoted by Cilento[7] referring to a promulgation made in 1844, it read —

> ... *we are absolutely certain about the accuracy of our hypothesis; that to* [every section of] *mankind is given a particular place by the Lord of Creation which is his Native Land, where all things are so placed as to suit him particularly, and thus preserve his race. He cannot trespass the length and breadth of this boundary without damage to his health, and danger to his life.*

The early twentieth century version of this came into full bloom under the guiding hand of Ellsworth Huntington of Yale, an influential American geographer who began his life's work about 1907. The following sums up Huntington's views fairly well —

> *The geographical distribution of health and energy depends on climate and weather, more than on any other single factor. The well known contrast between the energetic people of the most progressive parts of the temperate zone, and the inert inhabitants of the tropics and even of the intermediate regions such as Persia, is largely due to climate.*
>
> (Lee quoting Huntington)[8]

This was taken from Huntington's definitive work *Civilization and Climate.*[9] The corollary to this deterministic concept was postulation of a climate ideal for progress. Brown (1961)[10] stated that Huntington's views of this had produced an ideal climatic model rather akin to the climate of southern England and who, he asked, would regard London weather as perfection?

Obviously the implications of climatic determinism make it almost compulsory to believe that northern Europeans who attempted to settle permanently in the tropics would suffer "physical and moral degeneration".

To modern eyes this reads as extraordinary, but for those times it was a fair statement of the majority opinion. To many Englishmen of the nineteenth and early twentieth centuries even Australia was (with the exception of Tasmania) a hot sweaty place, the climate of which had a deleterious effect on the physique, mammary development and dentition of females, and was a cause of heat apoplexy and general deterioration in the male. Sydney in summer time was seen as a place for white suits and pith helmets and as a place in which the heat constantly tempted the unwary to excess indulgence in alcohol. (Harlin,[11] McCallum,[12] Editor, *A.M.G.,*[13] Griffiths[14]).

And, as for the real tropics, a century ago permanent settlement of such by Europeans was considered impossible. (Bolton[15]).

This view was supported by hard experience as the horrific death rates experienced by Europeans journeying to and residing in the tropics testified. (Consult Cilento & Lack,[16] Price,[17] Curtin,[18] Price,[19] Cilento,[20] Elkington[21] and Rodenwaldt[22]).

Curtin quotes Major Alexander Tulloch's official survey of mortality experience in the British Army, 1817–36.

	Deaths per 1000 p.a.
Among men of military age, civilians in U.K.	11.5
Same age group recruited into Army in U.K.	15.3
Service in Mediterranean zone and temperate North Africa	12– 20
Around tropical Indian Ocean (Mauritius, Ceylon)	30– 75
In troops in tropical America	85–138
In West Africa	483–668

In the days when Portugal and Spain were acquiring wide flung colonial territories only about 10 per cent of those who went to the Far East for a spell of service eventually lived to return home. (*See Endnote 1*)

All this seems to have very little relevance today, but it is just as well to realize that the *British Encyclopaedia* (1964 edition)[23] concluded the article on tropical medicine with the following:

> *Whether the white man can carve a permanent niche for himself and retain his faculties and stamina over generations, is still a moot question even after centuries of colonization. The answer awaits further experience under modern conditions and physiological research carried out in the tropical setting.*

And, even as late as 1945, an author who had not yet perceived how the new world was wagging, made a similar suggestion and proposed north east Australia as a suitable area for a trial of European colonization![24] Obviously he was a century too late.

Against this kind of background North Queensland was settled almost inadvertently without realization that it was in the tropics.

However, around the turn of the century, two happenings jolted Australia out of this kind of oblivious refusal to recognize heat when it was all around it.

The first factor had its origins outside Australia. Optimists, typified by Gorgas the distinguished medical officer who had created a healthy enclave for Europeans in the Panama zone, had begun to proclaim the potential for settlement of Europeans in tropical areas. The vast spaces of the Amazon basin, for example, would provide untold riches for colonists from an over populated Europe, so it was said. (In those days members of the master races did not have to worry over much about what indigenous peoples thought of such proposals.) However, such views put the climatic determinists on their mettle.

In the subsequent academic controversies an appeal to historical experience was made. What had, in fact, happened to European colonists who had tried to settle on tropical lowlands? This turned the spotlight on North Queensland since the people there, at that time (as I have mentioned already) seemed to be the only society of northern Europeans who had successfully made a *lowland* tropical area its home. Overseas experts greatly doubted that such a group of people existed, or if it did whether its members still possessed all their faculties, as it were. Cilento, Elkington and others were vigorous defenders of North Queensland man.

This debate was rather academic, though the emotions were sufficiently aroused to compel Elkington to make a troublesome journey to a remote island called Kissar in the Dutch East Indies to "prove" that a small isolated enclave of people descended from Dutch settlers many years before had retained their European characteristics. Nevertheless, these exchanges were hardly likely to arouse general interest in Australia.

The second happening, however, was a different kettle of fish. For somewhat different reasons the Australian working class and a certain number of people cast in the sensitive democratic mould were determined that if federation came to pass the Kanakas who had been indentured to work the sugar cane plantations in Queensland had to go back to their home islands. But Queensland interests demanded a price for a vote favourable to federation. The rest of

Australia would have to be prepared to subsidize financially a northern sugar industry worked with white labour only. The idea of a subsidy for a primary industry was absolutely anathema in those times and a great number of people who lived in southern states became highly emotional over the prospect of paying high domestic prices for sugar which could be imported cheaply.

Lofty philosophies excite men's minds mightily when they also stimulate their pockets. It was hoped that if it could be scientifically demonstrated that white men could not work and live efficiently in the tropics then those with over sensitive consciences and those who hated the threat of competition from black labour might become reconciled to having plantations worked by black labour. (After all, Queensland was not quite civilized, anyway!)

As it turned out, Australians did not have to pay extra for their sugar until 1923, and according to some interpretations, not till 1945.[25] And in any case, plantations and their Kanakas were being replaced steadily by individual white farmers even before all this occurred. (*See Endnote 2*)

But as a result of this fear of over costly domestic sugar, for at least twenty-five years our medical literature and our various medical meetings were full of the subject of the northern European's ability to adapt to tropical work and residence. As Atlee Hunt[26] the then Under-Secretary to the Department of External Affairs has since pointed out, it turned out to be a great ado about a subject which was of little importance:

> *The belief that the tropics were unhealthy, at any rate for men engaged in manual labour, had been sedulously cultivated by interested persons and that belief had an effect in deterring working men of white races from seeking manual work in the cane fields.*

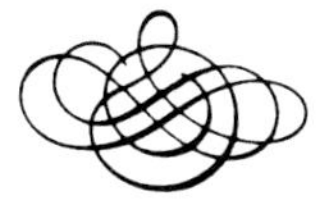

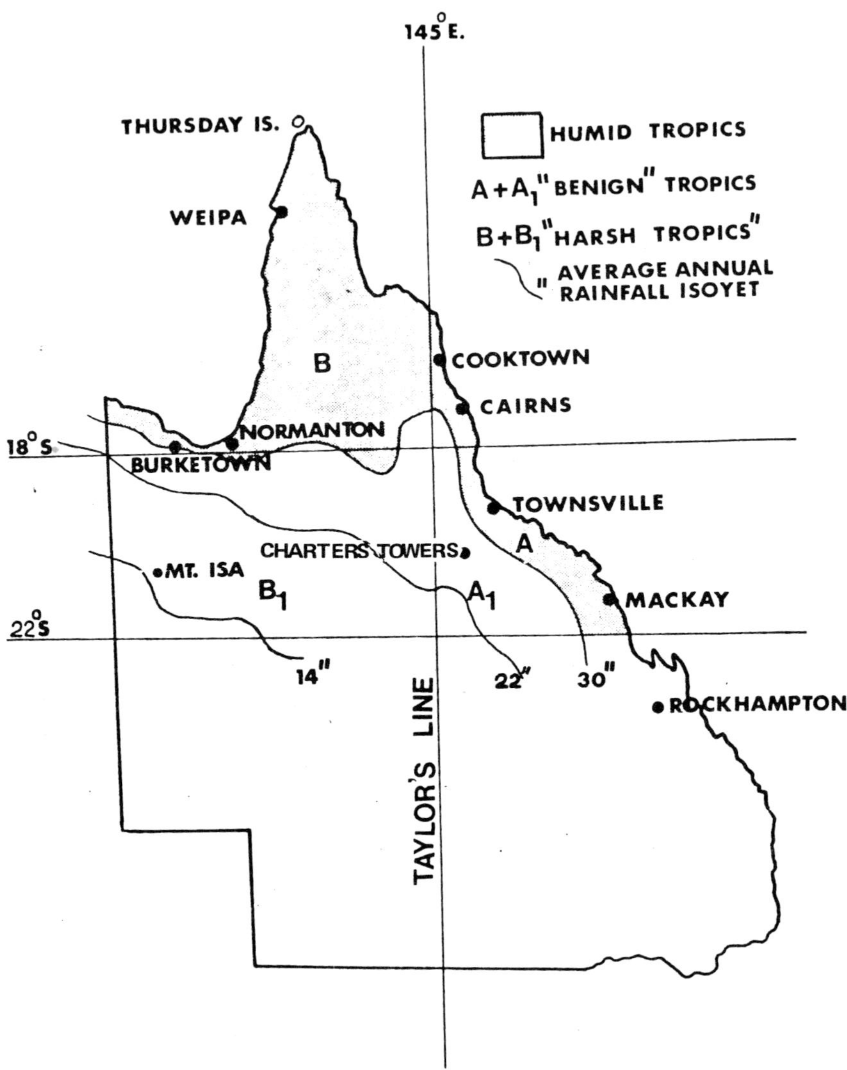

Figure 2:   *TROPICAL QUEENSLAND 10°S LAT. 22°S LAT.*

THE NORTH QUEENSLAND CLIMATE

At this stage there is an obligation to show that the North Queensland climate does produce those stresses usually associated with living in tropical lowlands.

In fact, experts such as Taylor[27] consider that the climate in northern Australia is a difficult one. He stated that the Australian coast from Cooktown to Broome contains some of the hottest places on earth — particularly Wyndham. He equated Broome with the mouth of the Congo; Darwin with Bathurst in West Africa; Alice Springs with Peshawar; and Townsville with Calcutta.

In order to determine what constitutes tropical Queensland I have duly consulted writings of Taylor,[28] Price,[29] Lee,[30] Cilento[31] and Macpherson[32] and the usages of practical experience as embodied in the scale of extra wages paid for working in hot areas of the state. These 'loadings' are written into the various industrial awards.[33]

As a result of this I have produced a tropical area as shown in *Fig. 2*. The tropical area lies north of 22°S lat. and is divided by a longitude 145°E long., which I have presumed to call Taylor's line after that great Australian geographer. To the west of this line are the 'harsh' tropics (Taylor) and to the east the benign tropics, my own description. Both areas contain wet and dry tropics.

Benign tropics (trade wind tropics)

Most of this area has a satisfactory to high reliable rainfall for eight months of the year, with south east trade winds particularly in autumn and winter. The wet season occurs in the first months of the year with cyclones from the east and north east. These cyclones usually do not cause much damage and they are compatible with sugar growing.[34]

The area is mainly lowlands with a few small usable plateaux — mainly around Atherton and Herberton. Most of the population live near the coast. In 1966 there were 260,000 people[35] and the majority had ready access to marine forms of recreation.

Germane to this the northern vector of malaria, *Anopheles faurati*, is efficient down to about 19°S latitude, which is in the vicinity of Townsville. Cairns is the only urban centre of any size in the area with a high potential for endemic malaria.

The summer climate on the Queensland coast does not vary greatly between Cairns and Rockhampton but there is a continuing gradation of difference in winter as one moves up the coast. In terms of climatic stress, Lee (1940)[36] equates Townsville with Mackay but Cairns with Cloncurry. Since the latter is several degrees of latitude south of Cairns but in the 'harsh' tropics, this judgment serves to illustrate the tougher conditions prevailing in the inland.

Harsh tropics

The harsh tropics are subject in varying degrees to the influence of the Asian–Australian monsoon which comes from the north west. The rainfall is unreliable in many districts and dry conditions prevail for nine months of the year. If the populations of Mt Isa, Weipa and Torres Straits are subtracted, then in 1966 approximately 20,000 people occupied 200,000 square miles.

Lee[37] considers that the climate in the Peninsula and Gulf, that is, the wet area of the harsh tropics, is very trying. The Gulf area always has been "heartbreak corner". Stokes[38] in 1841 viewed the great plains of dry grass almost in ecstasy and wrote that he —

> *... breathed a prayer that ere long the now level horizon would be broken by a succession of tapering spires rising from the Christian hamlets that must ultimately stud this country.*

The outcome was far different. In 1869 the depressed pastoral community around Burketown petitioned the Queensland Parliament to the effect:

> *... the treeless plains tortured the sheep in the summer heat, and in winter, no rains fell and the waterholes become sun-baked mud.*[39]

It is a truly harsh land with little capacity for primary industry. And its higher rainfall areas constituted the main malarial endemic areas in Queensland, that is, Torres Strait, "Gulf" and most of the "Peninsula".

Let us return to a consideration of the tropical area in general. The "shaded areas" on the map (*Fig. 2*) represent the wet tropics (approximately).[40]

This division of the environment under consideration must necessarily be arbitrary. Argument about boundaries is inevitable. Lee[41] has written:

> *The term 'tropical' must remain vague ... We all know in general fashion what is meant by a tropical climate. But wherever a dividing line is put, somebody will want it moved north, and somebody also will want it moved south.*

This sums up the fact that, in spite of gloomy predictions to the contrary, northern Europeans have made a truly tropical area their permanent home. It now remains to state my thesis, which purports to explain why this venture was carried out so successfully.

MY THESIS

Those who believed that white people could not successfully develop North Queensland without black labour, considered that tropical disease and climatic stress would be the most disastrous impediments to efficient settlement. Thus almost inevitable ill health and racial deterioration would prove to be almost insurmountable limiting factors.

My thesis would reject this and contend that during the period in which tropical Queensland was settled the most important influence favouring successful permanent settlement was the establishment of industries viable within the Australian economy. I would stress that these industries had to be profitable in terms of our standards of living. Thus, any industry must have been sufficiently affluent to have supported the local population within the standards of technology which were then developing.

Once this was achieved then health comparable to that found elsewhere in Queensland almost automatically followed. Thus, I put economically viable industry, and not health, as the first requirement necessary to establish successful settlement. This is not new. It was stated by Sir James Barrett in 1935:[42]

> *The conclusion reached is that white people do live and thrive in most parts of tropical Australia, where it is possible to conduct a profitable industry.*

And, it was said again by Brown[43] in 1961:

> *The problems of population in northern Australia are essentially problems connected with those of industrialisation in general.*

Price (1939)[44] remarked that:

> *... one feels that the primary factors are economic.*

A subsidiary thesis would be that most tropical diseases cease to be a major problem if there are the motives and the means to improve diet, to get rid of filth, to establish sound sanitation, to provide safe water, to promote personal cleanliness and to do something effective about mosquito breeding and mosquito contacts. (There are some obvious exceptions to this, particularly in Equatorial Africa.)

This sounds awfully like old fashioned public health, highly effective in any climate, which does not require sophisticated medical services. Motivation usually comes with improved education; and the "means" are provided by a sound economy. In fact the latter usually is a necessary basis for adequate universal education as well.

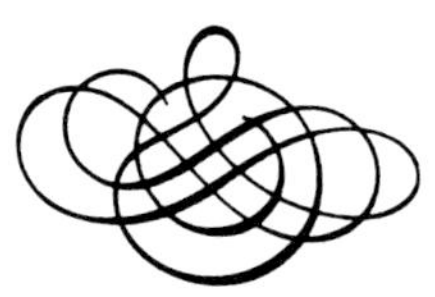

PART II

THE SOCIAL ENVIRONMENT

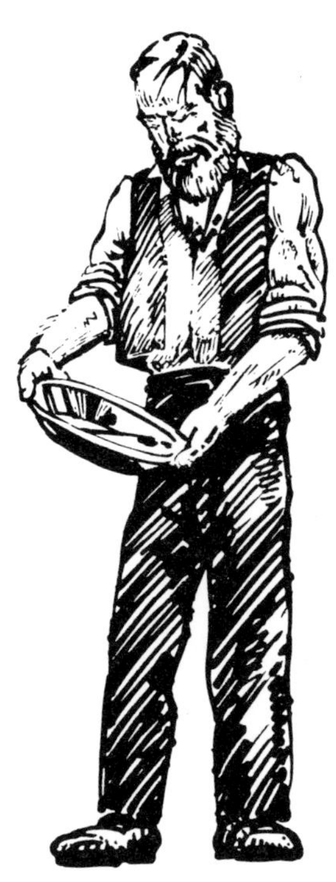

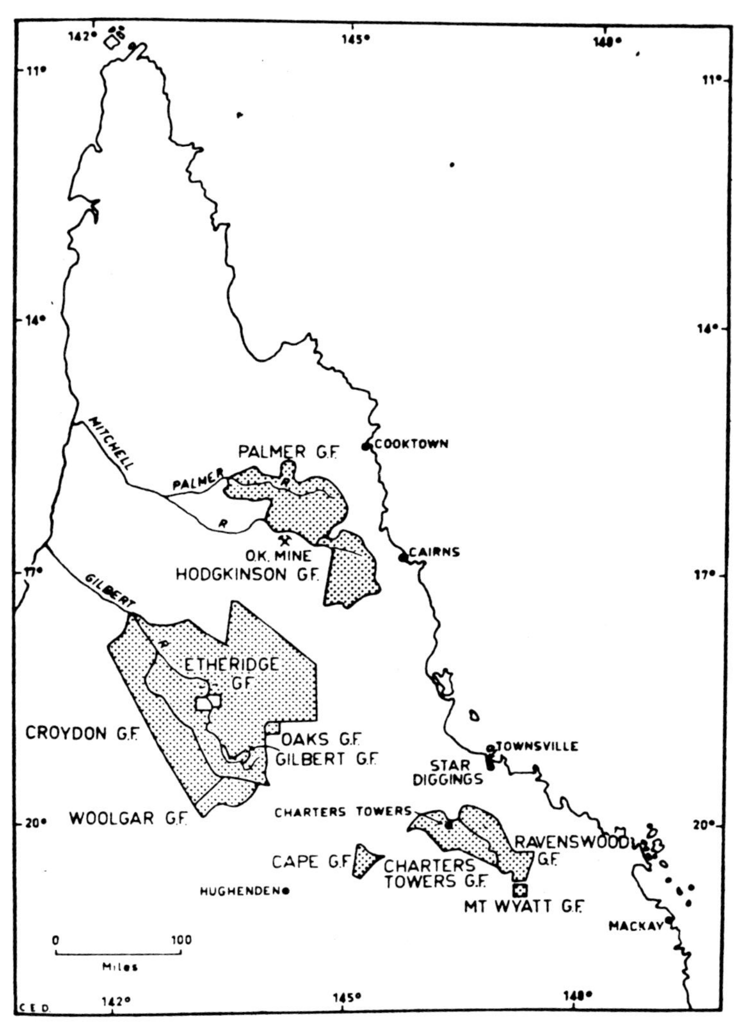

NORTH QUEENSLAND, AUSTRALIA,
SHOWING THE SITES OF THE
STATE'S PRINCIPAL GOLD FIELDS

14

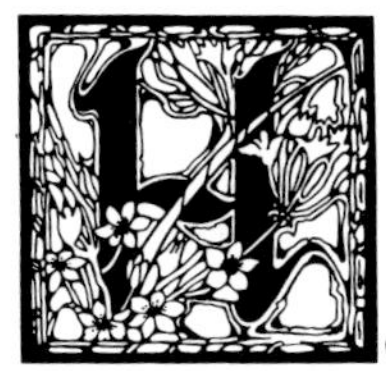ere I will discuss the following:

- The development in North Queensland of three major viable industries — pastoral, mining and sugar cane growing.

- The composition of the population and the manner in which it lived.

THE INDUSTRIES

In this discussion of industrial development I have not used primary sources to any extent. For industrial undertakings in the benign tropics I have leant heavily on G.C. Bolton's *A Thousand Miles Away*.[45]

For happenings in the Gulf I have consulted F.H. Bauer's *Historical Geographic Survey of Part of Northern Australia,* Part I, Introduction and the Eastern Gulf Region.[46] A number of reminiscences also were available. *Mines in the Spinifex* provided valuable information.[47]

After much trial and error three industries demonstrated an ability to survive in North Queensland, namely, pastoral, mining and sugar cane growing. And this has continued to the present day.

The value of primary production for tropical Queensland is listed as follows (1966–67):

1.	Sugar		$ 101,465,000	36.7%
2.	Mining		$ 83,921,000	30.3%
3.	Pastoral		$ 58,495,000	21.1%
	(Sheep & Wool	5.6%		
	Cattle	15.5%)		
4.	Forest Products		$ 3,123,000	1.1%
				89.2%

(Queensland Year Book)[48]

The pastoral industry

The search for pastoral land originally opened up the country. Sheep were first tried but did not do well. They have gradually been replaced by cattle, except in the central area of the drier parts of the north west.

Governor Bowen, contemplating the manner in which the northern lands were settled, saw —

> *... something almost sublime in the steady, silent flow of pastoral occupation over north-eastern Australia. It resembles the rise of the tide or some other operation of nature, rather than a work of man.*[49]

And Phillips (1903)[50] wrote of Edward Palmer:

> *... one of that brave band of pioneer squatters who in the early sixties swept across North Queensland with their flocks and herds, settling as if by magic, great tracts of hitherto unoccupied country, and thereby opening several new ports on the east coast and on the shores of the Gulf of Carpentaria, to the commerce of the world.*

However, there were slightly more ribald ideas about the quality of the early pioneers of the "Gulf":

> *God forsaken, devil may care,*
> *Every one with his sins to bear,*
> *From East, from West, they are company there*
> *Where all the bad lots go.*
>
> (Palmer)[51]

Unfortunately, there was no market for cattle and there also was a "depression" in the late sixties. But, beginning with the gold rush to the Cape River in 1867, the miners started pouring in and so provided local mouths to consume the beef until such time as freezing and canning techniques based on meatworks at Townsville,

Cairns and Bowen became a reality. Northern meat is not usually a gourmet's delight, but nevertheless it is successfully marketed around the world. The pastoral industry's survival represents shrewd adaptation to a fairly tough environment.

Mining

Most of the alluvial gold had been won by the end of the 1870s; deep mining began to decline in Charters Towers at the turn of the century; the real boom in other metals in the Herberton area was almost over by World War I. The copper mining in the far north west has proved to be a continuing story. And in later years, silver, lead and zinc (and later copper as well) have sustained Mt Isa. But at the turn of the century mining in North Queensland was starting to decline, though at the time, this was not recognized. The point is that this falling off in mining happened after Federation when the sugar growers had to gradually repatriate the Kanaka labour force. Thus, an acclimatized, intelligent white labour force of ex-miners became available to take their place. (In more recent times the mining of alumina, vast quantities of coal and less successfully nickel is assuring the affluent continuation of a tropical mining industry.)

Sugar growing

As the sugar cane plantations gave way to sugar cane farms and as the Kanakas gradually departed, the decrease in gold mining thus indirectly tended to make the sugar industry highly efficient. A number of miners in the original 'rushes' to North Queensland were mature men who had battled through every 'rush' since those on the western coast of North America in 1849. They and their successors were adventurous, fiercely independent and heartily disliked working for wages. They helped develop a northern tradition. Their backgrounds were diverse and in some cases quite cosmopolitan. These men had a political awareness, a social perception and an experience of life which was the reverse of that of the southern 'cocky' farmer. (Nothing addles a lad's natural curiosity quicker than pressing his head against a cow's flank, hand milking twice a day.)

A remarkable primary industry was created, sited on pockets of rich soil up and down the narrow coastal plains which lie between the mountains and the sea. Very early on it was an industry which became highly organized (and regimented) with complex co-operative and marketing structures. The very criticism which sugar growing attracted from the southern states of Australia goaded it to establish quite sophisticated research institutes studying the breeding of canes, farming techniques and milling. It generally is conceded that it is the most efficient cane sugar industry in the world in terms of production per acre and in the efficiency of extraction of sugar from cane. (However, its product is not the cheapest. Only in certain periods has our sugar been globally competitive in price.)

Cedar getting

Forestry products in terms of money cannot be compared with the three major industries in North Queensland but a brief mention should be made of the timber industry, if only for one reason. In all the questioning that went on in the first two decades of this century about the capacity of white men to work hard under hot, humid conditions, no one seemed to remember the cedar getters. In the early years of settlement, these rather isolated men were usually the first to work through the steaming rain forests which grew on the narrow coastal plains. One can hardly imagine harder work under more trying conditions; and yet, judging by the way the cedar was rapidly depleted, they performed their task all too successfully! (I have found only one reference to their health — to the effect that they suffered the same fevers as the aborigines.) (Clarke)[52]

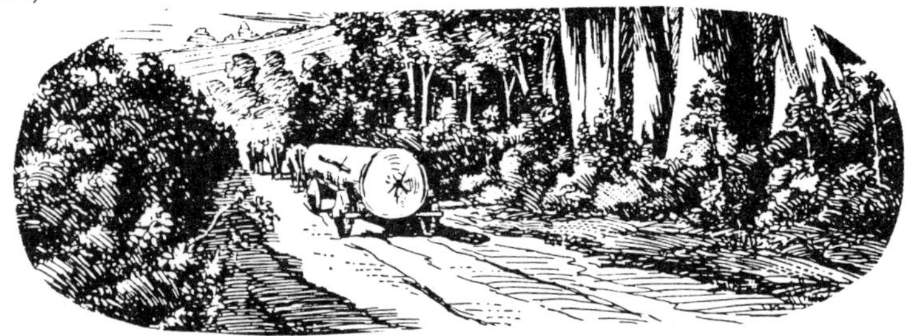

The work force

I must now revert to the calibre of the work force because I think this was important in North Queensland development. Its members have shown quite a deal of initiative both in industry and politics. It probably was no accident that the great shearers' strike of 1891 started at Barcaldine in western Queensland on the edge of the tropics, that in its heyday the north and the west rather than the city proletariat was the backbone of the Labor Party, and that much of the racist bitterness which engendered the "White Australia" policy stemmed from the turmoil with the Chinese on the Palmer River.

Unlike the more closely settled farming areas such as the Darling Downs which voted solidly against Federation[53] the work force in the outlying areas mainly was in favour of it.

In this century the tropical electorates have produced a succession of state premiers and several federal leaders such as Theodore and Fadden.

The labours of these miners created the phenomenon of Charters Towers, in its heyday a permanent tropical city of at least 22,000 people, the largest outside Brisbane. It had a Stock Exchange and a School of Mines. The latter produced 'graduates' a decade before there was a university in Queensland. Its citizens called it "The World" and felt they enjoyed amenities and educational facilities superior to any others in the colony. As indeed probably they did. Due to their mining and commercial interests they had contacts with a wider world outside Australia. (The amount of English capital sunk in holes in the ground in those parts was prodigious.) Charters Towers was proclaimed a municipality in June 1877.[54]

Much the same could be said about the initiative and courage of the medical practitioners who practised in North Queensland. No doubt some were seeking their own particular brand of oblivion at land's end, but the majority were alert men, keenly interested in the strange medical problems which they encountered. There was a North Queensland Medical Society early on;[55] North Queenslanders were well represented at the early Intercolonial Medical Congresses and about a dozen papers were published by northern practitioners before the turn of the century, including one which does not usually appear in bibliographies collected by subsequent writers, viz., Salter's description of maladies suffered by pearl divers at Thursday Island.[56] At the Australasian Medical Congress held in Adelaide in 1905 Dr T.R. MacDonald of Innisfail (then Geraldton) read a paper on "Medicine and Sociology" — surely ahead of its time.

One should remember also Walter Edmund Roth, one of three brothers, sons of a London surgeon, all of whom have received mention in the *Australian Encyclopaedia*. In 1894 he went as a hospital superintendent in turn to Boulia, Cloncurry and Normanton Hospitals. These names do not suggest an environment which would stimulate research. Yet in 1897 he published his *Ethnological Studies Among North-West Central Aborigines.* Shortly afterwards he became Protector of Aboriginals for North Queensland. He later went to British Guyana where he established a reputation as a prominent English anthropologist.[57] So much for the quality of the early work force in North Queensland.

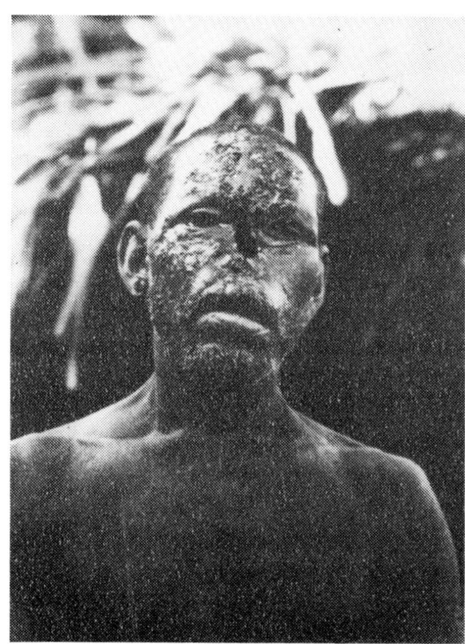

Health problems among Torres Straits Islanders. Tissue destruction by a non-syphilitic spirochete which causes Yaws and Framboesia. In this instance the manifestation was called Gangosa and was easily confused with Leprosy.

The aboriginal population

The presence of an indigenous population which was nomadic in habit and not far along the scale of social development, made its partial cruel destruction, dispersal and subsequent brutal subjugation relatively easy. Industries could thus develop as they wished without let or hindrance from a culture already long in residence.

And this affected health in three ways. White people had to do many menial and manual tasks; a native population did not serve as a reservoir of infection for a variety of communicable diseases — in fact it was the other way around. We gave them our own ill health. And when the time came to effect improvement by changing the environment — sanitation, personal hygiene etc. — the relatively homogeneous population of European origin was much more amenable to this kind of change than a culturally complex indigenous population would have been.

We now know, as well, a fact which a few people had been suggesting for a long time. That is, that tropical adaptation occurs more readily and efficiently if the newcomer has to carry out a reasonable degree of strenuous physical activity. In other words, the social group which has to do its own work from street cleaning up to the higher flights of administration, has more chance of successful adaptation. Furthermore, Haran at Cape York made the astonishing statement that the only disability suffered by the detachment of marines at the Port of Refuge was due to 'rheumatism' and bronchitis.[58,59,60] At that period there apparently was very little transference of communicable diseases from the indigenous people.

The three major industries not only were established successfully but were maintained in a financially viable state, often by complementing each other and providing mutual support. This paper contends that economic and social stability which resulted from this supplied the motivation and means to improve diet and housing, to provide sanitation and to encourage personal cleanliness. In addition, the establishment of schools, hospitals and clinical medical services was justified by the presence of a community which obviously was financially sound.

And as a result of this, health hazards were overcome. (*See Endnote 3*)

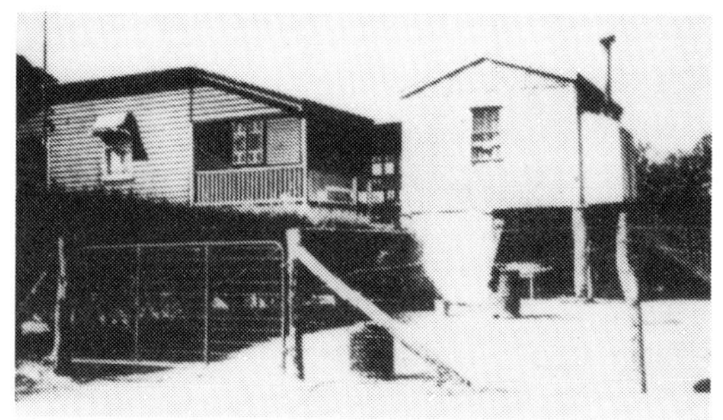

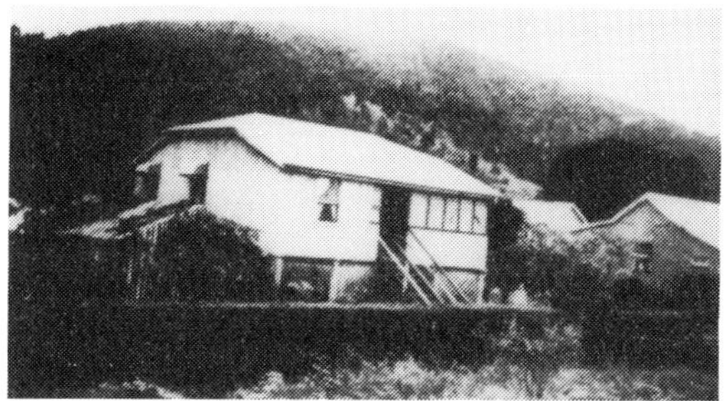

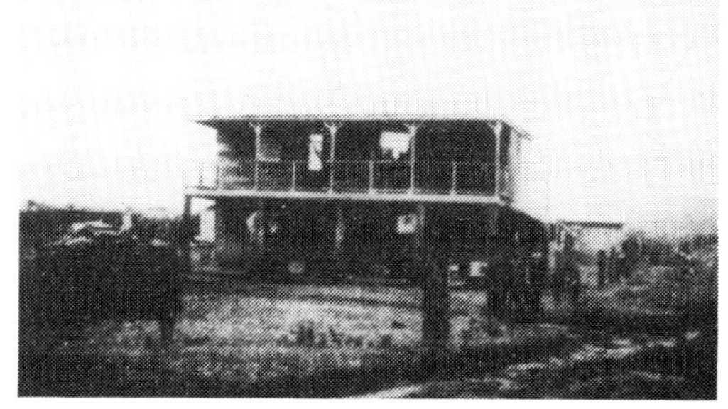

HOW PEOPLE LIVED IN NORTH QUEENSLAND
c. 1920
These homes were small and hot. In the top picture, a galvanised iron annexe has been added to the house.

THE WAY PEOPLE LIVED

There is no doubt that the physical environments in which people lived were conducive to disease — particularly the filth diseases. When a new district was being opened up or when a mining field was being developed, people lived in tents or bark shanties and used water from a nearby creek or waterhole. Waste disposal — particularly faecal — was random and haphazard. Fly breeding was thus encouraged and water contamination became a likely event. Thus typhoid, dysentery and other bowel infections of less serious import were commonplace. In the coastal areas of North Queensland there was an added numerically minor hazard — scrub typhus — when rain forest was being cleared for cultivation.

Therefore, permanent settlement usually brought an improvement in health, but even so most people even then lived meagrely and under dirty conditions. Families were large and over-crowded into small houses. In the Queensland colony at that time — sixties and seventies — a woman who married in her early twenties went on to produce, on average, a completed family of eight babes.

There were many unmarried men and for them alcoholism and venereal disease were obvious threats. However, whether North Queensland settlements were dirtier and more unhealthy than towns in other parts of the colony would be a matter for debate.

We do know however, how people lived in the early 20th century in the tropical parts of the new State. (Queensland ceased to be a colony with Federation.) In the early twenties there was a magnificent piece of sociological research carried out by a nurse, Miss Gorman, under Raphael Cilento's direction. She closely investigated the manner of living in 740 families — in Townsville (300), Cairns (123), Charters Towers (132), Julia Creek (24), on the Atherton Tableland (81) and in Cloncurry (80). There was a bias towards lower socio-economic households. When much that has been written since has been forgotten, the results of this survey will still be studied.[61]

The 'ordinary' townsfolk lived meanly, as they did in Brisbane at that time, in hot little wooden houses — sometimes lacking a water supply in the kitchen, sometimes in unceiled and poorly lighted rooms and sometimes with deficient facilities for bathing. The houses often were close together — three to four feet apart. A minority had dirt floors. Most houses had a 'wood' stove, sometimes in addition to a gas one, since for culinary achievement housewives had no faith in gas stoves.

Of more relevance to health, food storage often was deficient. Thirty percent had no ice chests, 40% no meat safes — meat often hung on hooks in a roofed but open gangway where there was a cool draught. (This was the custom in our household. The 'meat safe' occupied such a place.)

A Prague geographer visited North Queensland in 1910 and reported:

> *... the indulgence in intoxicating liquors, especially in those of very bad quality; the consumption of meat one and the same kind — in a 'state that baffles description'; the scant supply of fruit and vegetables and the bad water supply, are all important factors in inducing a condition of ill-health.*[62]

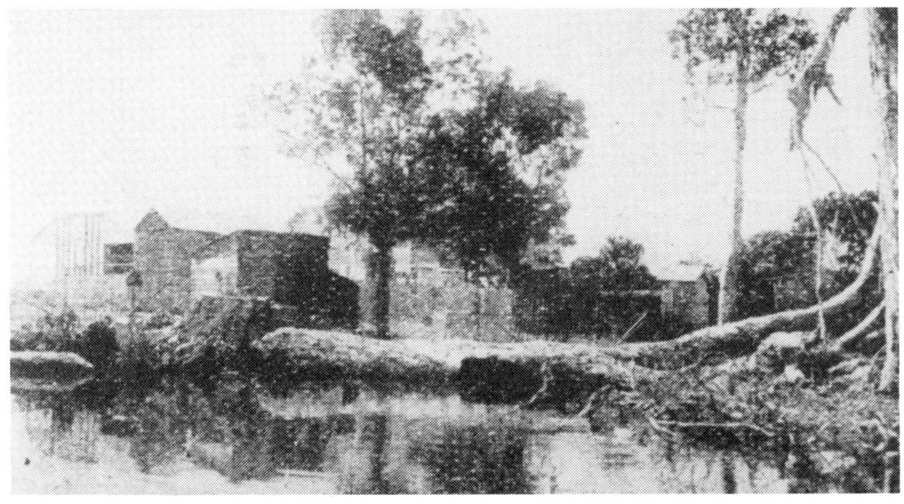

Poor water supplies and poor drainage were a problem in pioneering days in the tropical north. This photograph shows a swamp beside a domestic dwelling in Cairns, circa 1910-1920.

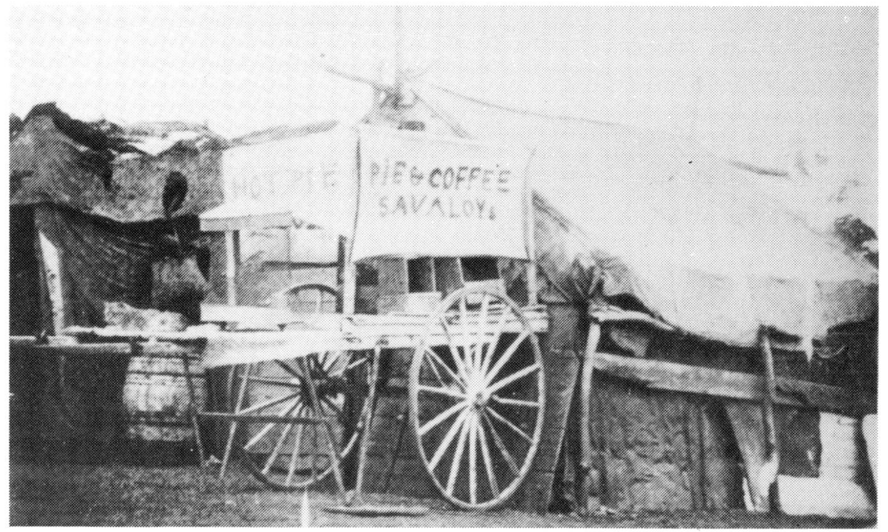

Coffee and Pie Cart, North Queensland.
Obvious deficiencies in hygiene.

The advent of plague in 1900 focussed attention on environmental sanitation. Later, the survey carried out by the Australian Hookworm Campaign had a similar effect. The survey produced the following information about toilet facilities in North Queensland:

37,837 premises were inspected.
15.6% of the toilets were up to standard.
81.6% of the toilets were defective.
2.8% of the premises had no toilet facilities.[63]

The Annual Reports of the Commissioner of Public Health and particularly the illustrations therein, are extremely informative. We learn from the 1908 Report that one section of Malaytown in Cairns was so beyond redemption that it was burnt down. It was stated in the 1904 Report that 360 loads of filth were removed from Cairns, and 2000 loads from Townsville. In the latter city, much to the annoyance of the Public Health Commissioner, water drawn from near the outlet of the sewer was used to lay the dust on the streets.[64]

The milk supply sometimes was deficient in quantity and poor in quality, and in some households milk was not available. Foodstuffs were transported and retailed under circumstances which would provoke reactions of horror today.[65]

Cilento had written in 1925:

> *It is not uncommon to find that the water supply is polluted, inadequate and fails to reach any recognized standard of desirability. ... that the milk supply is inferior and in amount trifling and variable. Greens may be almost unprocurable because people will not grow them.*

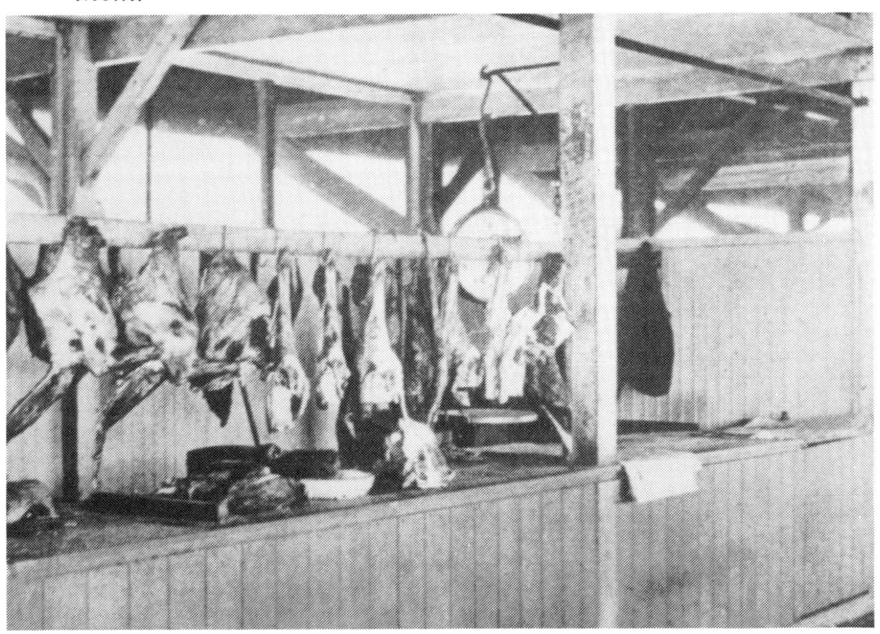

A well-ventilated butcher's shop in a north Queensland town, circa 1920.

Tanks were unscreened, drainage was non-existent or defective and collections of water abounded. In many towns and townships there were times of drought when the communal water supply became suspect. However, there is also no doubt that much the same might have been found in many other parts of Queensland.[66, 67]

In January 1919, Waite, the original American medical officer in Queensland, from the International Health Board of the Rockefeller Foundation, was invalided home with sprue. Lambert, an American who took over, remarked jocularly that in his rather short period as Director of the Queensland Hookworm Campaign until October 1919, he had supervised the building of over 4000 model latrines and the repair of 4000 more.[68] He was impressed with the vigour and drive of the local population in getting things done, once they were persuaded that they should be done.

These descriptions have been given to bring home the point that even in living memory Queenslanders lived in a spartan and dirty way. It was obvious that a good clean up would work wonders.

However, good protein from beef was in plentiful supply and quite cheap by the standard of the times. When preparing this paper I interviewed the Administrator of the School of Public Health and Tropical Medicine in Sydney. As a lad he had started his clerical career at the Australian Institute of Tropical Medicine in Townsville. He related how he always had meat for the morning and evening meals, but in addition he 'biked' home every lunch hour to a large steak which his mother grilled on top of the 'wood' stove.

Ethnic origins

It has been claimed that in actual fact North Queensland was not settled by northern Europeans but by southern Europeans, namely, Italians. I have consulted a number of sources. (*See Refs. 69, 70, 71, 72, 73*). We [the Department of Social and Preventive Medicine] learned as well quite a deal about the population of certain districts in North Queensland when doing field surveys to determine skin cancer prevalence. My conclusions are as follows:

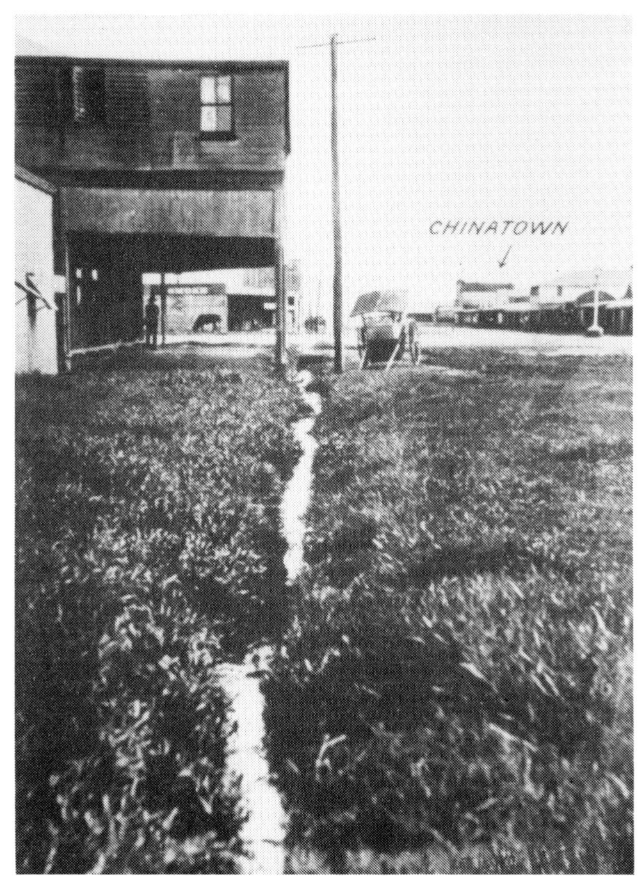

*Poor drainage was compounded by the problems of the
seasonal monsoon in coastal areas of North Queensland.
This photograph shows stagnating open drains,
overgrown with grass, in Cairns.
Chinatown, the ethnic centre for many who remained
after the gold rushes, is in the background, right.*

The Italian migration took place mainly in the 20th century and particularly after World War I. They settled chiefly in sugar growing areas north of Townsville where their descendants now form not a majority but a substantial minority of the population. North Queensland settlement had become a viable entity before these migrants had arrived.

Population mobility

It also is stated that the population of North Queensland always had been a mobile one — people moving up from southern states to "get a quick quid" — and then moving back again. It is difficult to find evidence about this subject. What evidence we do have suggests that the true tropical population is less than is usually surmised.

I have fallen back on Cilento's survey of many years ago[61] which was mainly urban, and our own surveys for skin cancer, which were mainly rural.[70] (We were interested only in people on the electoral rolls — that is, twenty-one years and over.)[74] My tentative guess would be that at least a third to half of the total tropical population at any one time has come from outside the tropics. If adults only were being considered, probably only about a third of the present population has been born in tropical Queensland. [In the total present population of Australia about one-sixth has been born outside Australia.][75]

The fact that tropical Queensland is not a foreign country but part of continental Australia probably has greatly assisted in its settlement. A period of work can be tried there without the necessity to migrate to another country; no formalities are required and no work permits are needed. This has led to self-selection of a work force which likes living in a hot climate. And the reverse applies as well. Those born in North Queensland who do not like residing there can just as easily depart for other parts of Australia.

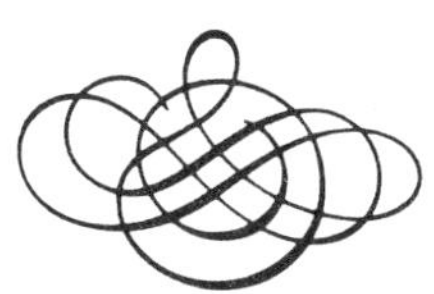

PART III

DISEASES AND EFFECTS OF CLIMATIC STRESS

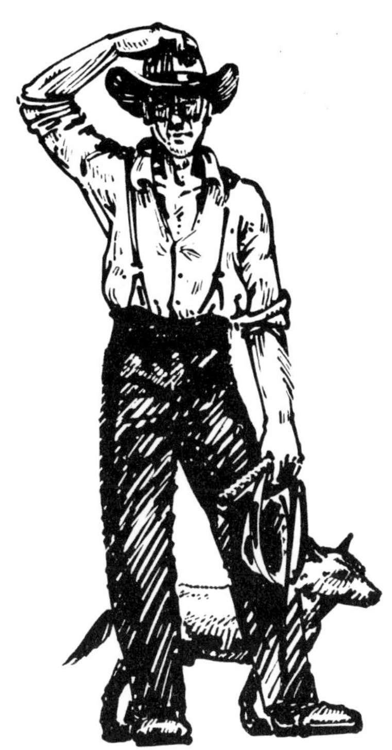

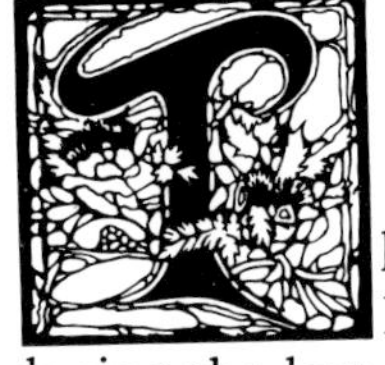his part discusses the diseases which afflicted the European settlers in North Queensland, particularly during the last four decades of the nineteenth century.

Taken in conjunction with the climatic stress previously described, would a potential settler have been deterred from setting up a permanent home in the area and rearing children therein? No doubt, what the settler thought of the obvious social disadvantages, such as isolation, would have influenced the family's decision.

The question is not what we, as medical practitioners of the present day, think of the matter but what the North Queensland layman thought about these things fifty to one hundred years ago. There was, of course, Byron's views on the effect of hot climates:

> *What men call gallantry, and gods adultery,*
> *Is much more common where the climate's sultry.*

> (Don Juan's Canto I, Stanza 63)

PATTERNS OF DISEASE

The problems caused by sickness in North Queensland have to be looked at relative to such problems elsewhere in the colony. In the sixties and seventies in Queensland approximately 50 per cent of all deaths occured in babes and children in the first five years of life, because, due to high fertility, a large proportion of the population was young, and because there were high death rates in the first five years of life, especially in the first year which was called infancy. The school child had the healthiest period in the total life span. Adolescence and young adulthood experienced much risk. Only 10 per cent of all deaths were in people fifty years and over. Those 65 years and over made up only 1% to 2% of the population in all Australia.

Compared with England at this period Australia had a higher death rate due to accidents and a somewhat lower one due to diseases caused by microbes.

TABLE I

Infant Mortality Rates*

Period	Brisbane	Tropical Queensland	Darling Downs (approx.)
1866–1875	145	137	114
1876–1885	180	140	106
1886–1895	145	123	76
1896–1905	128	99	84
1906–1915	90	64	63 [†]

* Number of infants who died in the first year of life per 1000 live births.
[†] Not precisely the same area as in the previous periods.

TABLE 2

Number of Births per Period in the Areas Stated

Period	Brisbane	Tropical Queensland	Darling Downs (approx.)
1866–1875	14981	3270	6954
1876–1885	15348	11561	10595
1886–1895	22066	26913	11583
1896–1905	18792	26279	13307
1906–1915	31001	30668	23671 [†]

[†] Not precisely the same area as in the previous periods.

Infant mortality rates

A medical demographer seeking data which will enable him to assess health almost automatically turns to infant mortality. (Fortunately it is a statistic which does not require an accurate diagnosis of cause of death; and it also tends to mirror prevailing socio-economic conditions.) Infant mortality is the number of deaths in the first year of life per 1000 live births.

Infant mortality rates were not available for each district of the colony[76, 77] but the number of deaths 0–2 years and the number of births were. As well as this I could obtain the ratio of number of deaths in the first year of life to number of deaths in the second year of life for the colony as a whole year by year.[78] Hence a fairly accurate estimate of district infant mortality rates can be made. This I did. The resulting information is set out in Tables 1 and 2. An infant born in tropical Queensland had a better chance of surviving until his first birthday than one born in Brisbane. This was to be expected since the cities were more unhealthy than the country centres until the 1920s. However, Darling Downs was healthier than North Queensland — also not unexpected.

Henry Jordan, that very perceptive early Registrar–General (Q) remarked:

> *As the general condition of the healthfulness or otherwise is, perhaps, in almost all cases fatihfully reflected by the mortality of young children ...* [79]

> *... Where many children are born, many children die, because young life is always feeble and easily extinguished.* [80]

Around this period the approximate infant mortality rates prevailing in England and Wales were 150–160. In the seventies in London they were about 160; in Leeds, 205; and in Liverpool, 238.[81] Therefore, as far as infant health went, tropical Queensland demonstrated reasonable performance if judged by the standards of the times.

Diseases

After reading a number of definitive papers and reports[82 – 92] one can give an outline of the diseases which had some degree of specific connection with hot climates and which were present in tropical Queensland. The more common ones were dysentery (bacterial) which produced serious diarrhoea and 'fever'. The latter was a hotch potch including malaria, but the most important cause was typhoid. There also were two other filth diseases, hookworm and ophthalmia.

Then there were certain diseases connected with deficiencies in diet such as sprue, beri-beri, barcoo rot and barcoo spew. These occurred from time to time, yet they could not be said to pose a heavy burden numerically.

Dengue[92a] (in epidemics), filariasis, plague and leprosy were as prevalent, but even more so in southern Queensland than in tropical Queensland. Among the native people living in Torres Strait there were pudendal ulcers and a fearsome looking condition called gangosa.[92b, 92c] The hot climate encouraged a higher incidence of common skin conditions including skin cancer.

Alcoholism was a burden carried by the pioneers in all parts of the colony, but its ravages in a predominantly male society living under unstable social conditions in a hot climate were particularly excessive.

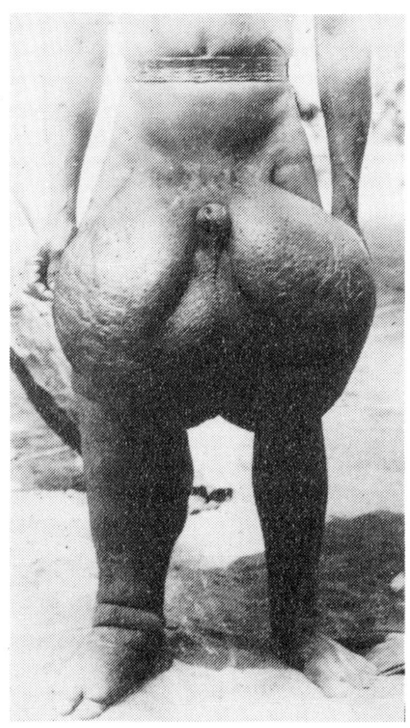

Health problems in the Torres Straits Islanders — a further example of Gangosa.

Fever and dysentery

The diseases most likely to kill and to frighten potential settlers away were the various 'fevers' and serious diarrhoeal disorders (dysentery). This probably has been the case in most tropical areas where Europeans have been badly mauled by disease. For example, Cilento and Lack[93] mention that of 951 deaths in Bengal, 573 were due to bowel infections and 268 to 'fevers'.

On the Palmer River gold rush in 1875, 28 people died of dysentery, 63 of 'remittent fever, fever etc.' and 2 of typhus fever. In Cooktown, 22 died of dysentery, 73 of 'remittent fever, fever etc.' and 9 of typhus fever. In the whole Queensland colony that year, 230 people died from 'remittent fever, fever etc.'. (I have used the nosological entry set down by the Registrar–General.)

The three disease entities in this group which were of numerical importance in tropical Queensland and which were potentially lethal were malaria, dysentery and typhoid. Typhoid predominated. Although a bowel infection, typhoid did not present with diarrhoea. It was a long drawn out fever.

Categorization

There were, however, great difficulties with categorization. There was, for instance, difficulty in separating malaria, typhoid and typhus (scrub and tick, not the classical louse type).[94, 95, 96, 97] Hence a diagnosis 'typho–malaria' was sometimes used, even though as early as 1849 the London fever hospital had made the necessary distinction between typhoid and louse typhus.[98] Sometimes, 'intermittent' was used for tertian malaria and 'remittent' for malignant malaria.[99] (*See Endnote 4*)

Early in this century it was realised that among the fevers there were entities other than typhoid and malaria. Terms such as coastal fever, Sarina fever, Mossman fever etc. were used. We now know that in the high rainfall areas on the coast, leptospirosis (in the sugar cane industry) and scrub typhus are not uncommon. There is an occasional patient with tick typhus and a few with murine typhus connected with maize growing on the Atherton Tableland.

Dengue tended to come in epidemics all over the colony and no doubt some patients with 'fever' were suffering from common viral conditions such as influenza.

Dysentery was common in tropical Queensland in the 19th century, particularly in mining camps, and the rush to the Palmer River probably witnessed the worst and most sustained outbreaks of fevers and diarrhoeal diseases. (In this century dysentery does not seem to have been a common diagnosis.)[100]

Morbidity from fevers and dysentery

It adds some drama to local medical history to believe, as is frequently stated, that certain railway lines in the Cairns–Mourilyan area produced one fever death for every sleeper laid during the course of construction. However, as is often the case, the truth is a drab creature. The incidence of 'fever' was high, its effects a continuing but apparently accepted burden and local epidemic incidents not infrequent.[104 – 106]

However, with the exception of certain dramatic happenings from time to time, the case fatality rate usually was generally low. For instance, Clarke[107] in 1913 stated that during the preceding five years in the Mossman area there had been 1482 fever patients with a case fatality rate less than 1%.

Hardie[108] in 1893 carried out a massive survey of admissions to hospitals in all districts throughout Queensland. Fever patients were found right throughout Queensland but were particularly frequent in the Cairns–Cooktown and Gulf areas. In the period 1887–91, 43% of all admissions to Cairns Hospital were on account of fevers. (I will comment later about death rates on the Palmer River.)

Hunt in 1892[109] studied the last 1000 patients admitted to Hughenden Hospital. He, like Hardie, combined all 'fevers' into one entity. Here are admissions due to fever expressed as a percentage of all admissions:

1887	1888	1889	1890	1891	1892
35.2%	30.1%	20.9%	15%	19.1%	8.5%

Hunt used these statistics to demonstrate that, as a district was stocked up, fever became less. It is rather difficult to know what these percentages signify in an area where a large proportion of the population consisted of single men without homes. This necessitated more frequent hospital admissions than would occur in a more stable community, where a man had womenfolk to look after him when he was sick. There is no doubt, however, that morbidity due to fever was high and that it occurred in 'dry' areas of the tropics such as Hughenden as well as in the wetter coastal areas.

However, in reading the outpourings of the various northern correspondents accredited to the *Brisbane Courier* (1875), one cannot help but be impressed by the *sang-froid* with which they viewed morbidity due to fevers etc.[110, 111, 112]

The most cryptic comment as the year drew to a close was:

... the public health of Cooktown is still depressed.[113]

(In this Cooktown epidemic, which began on 16th November, one suspects typhoid, since the water supply was said to be contaminated and it was the dry period of the year.)

The morbidity was looked at in terms of the time. The whole colony was subject to fevers and deaths from infectious disease. It was part of life, just as ischaemic heart disease, strokes, cancers and road deaths are part of life today. North Queensland was just a bit worse, but in this respect its citizens pointed out they had far less respiratory disease.

In the Landsborough Papers there is an unsigned letter (1866) to that rather scared pro-consul who had cautiously investigated the fever outbreak at Burketown and then hastily shifted his head-quarters to Sweer's Island. I believe the handwriting is that of Governor Bowen. The relevant section of the letter reads:

The temporary sickness which has occurred is said to
be common to all new settlements in the North; and it is
probable that it will cease when the countryside has
been fully occupied.[114]

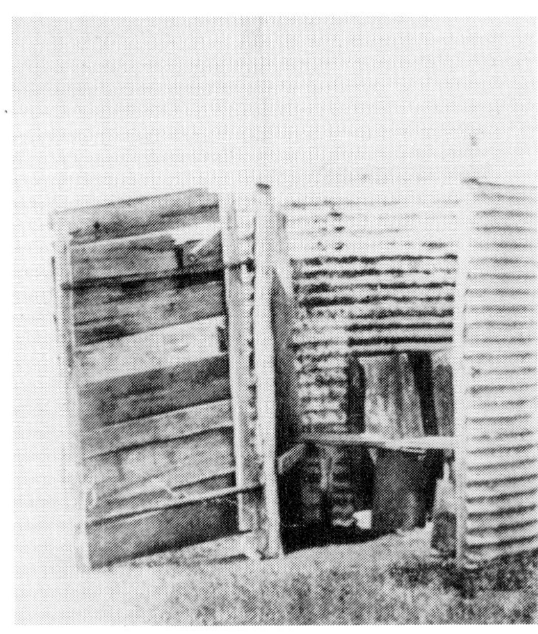

A Shire Councillor's earth closet, in Cairns, c. 1920.

A case of neglected "Example is better than precept."

Typhoid and dysentery were major causes of death in the development of North Queensland. Thirty-two percent of deaths were due to bowel infections prior to 1883. The figure had fallen to 9 percent by 1923, four decades later. These two photographs show the primitive state of sanitation still present in the 1920s.

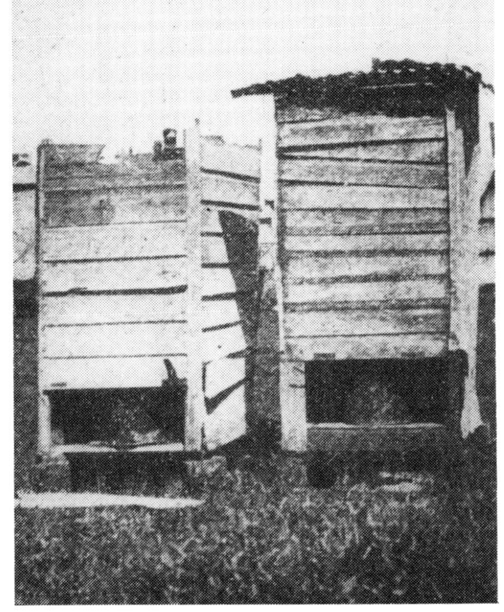

"State-of-the-Art" earth closets, North Queensland.

It was then suggested to Landsborough that he should move back to the mainland. As a comment on an epidemic of fever which had allegedly wiped out half a township, it does smack somewhat, by modern standards, of almost psychotic lack of feeling. But these were not modern days.

The best personal account of a prolonged bout of northern fever which I have read was penned by a gentle Dutch migrant who was the anonymous author of *Missing Friends 1871-1890.*[115] We now know him to have been T.P.L. Weitemeyer.[116]

Mortality from fever and dysentery

In the main the case fatality rate from 'fevers', typhoid, malaria etc. was not high. (We already have noted Clarke's statement about the Mossman district which is a little north of Cairns.) This tends to be confirmed by Derrick's definitive survey of North Queensland fevers (1957).[117]

Mitchell carried out a survey of deaths which had occurred in the Townsville Hospital between 1865 and 1923.[118] (However, that hospital area provides services for a somewhat drier area of North Queensland than does Cairns, or did Cooktown in its heyday.) He was able to find records of 12066 deaths — not including gastro-enteritis in children.

Causes of death which might in some way be deemed as part of living in the tropics accounted for only 1028 deaths; thus:

TABLE 3

Number of Deaths ('tropical' causes)
Townsville District, 1865–1923

Typhoid	570	Sprue	18
Dysentery	321	Dengue	52
		Malaria	61
		Filariasis	6
	891		**137**

41

Once again we see the importance of the bowel infections, particularly in a drier area where water supplies tended to become scarce in the last half of each year. When the number of deaths due to all types of infective intestinal disease including gastro-enteritis in children were expressed as a percentage of all deaths, Mitchell found that this ranged from 32.4 per cent in 1874–1883 to 8.7 per cent in 1914–1923. This gives an indication of how environmental sanitation — water supplies and removal of wastes — and personal hygiene had improved.

There were, however, certain outbreaks, usually isolated in time and place in which case fatality rates were high.

At Burketown in 1866 something like fifty people died. The population at risk might be considered as the population of the township itself — seventy odd; or of the district — perhaps 200 people. Elkington (1912) considered this to have been due to malignant malaria.[119] More data has now become available: Landsborough papers in the Oxley Library; the Landsborough 'Field Books' in Mitchell Library; files in the Government Archivist's Office (Brisbane) re Albert River. These throw a somewhat different light on events, but it still is very difficult to decide whether the deaths were due to malaria or typhoid.[120, 121] Considering the high fatality rate it was probably malignant malaria. I doubt if typhoid fever would have been so lethal.

Malaria (ex New Guinea) was introduced to the mining settlement of Kidston in 1910. There were 400 people; 120 went down with malaria and there were 24 deaths.[122] It is of interest to note that official medical positions in Queensland have had an unfortunate experience with 'fevers'. Ballow died of typhus in 1850;[123] Wray died of plague in 1902;[124, 125] and Zeitz, a local authority medical officer (part-time) died of typhoid at Cloncurry in 1913.[126]

Cairns has had epidemics of malaria periodically between 1881 and 1942. Quite a number of deaths occurred as a result of these but, in the main, tertian rather than malignant types of the disease tended to prevail. The 1942 (war time) epidemic (600–700 patients) was 'benign' in nature.

In the Sarina district between 1915 and 1922 Derrick points

out that there were 100 patients who suffered from 'Sarina fever' and 19 of them died. The epidemic of leptospirosis which occured at Ingham in 1933 ushered in the 'modern period' in which that fever became associated with cane cutting. There was then a considerable case fatality rate which has not been repeated in subsequent outbreaks.[127, 128, 129]

The Palmer River gold rush was a chaotic affair. It started in the summer of 1873–74 and continued on during the 1870s. It was mainly alluvial mining with no permanent settlement. Chinese miners were in a large majority. (For a lurid account read *River of Gold*).[130]

It was rare, however, for a death to occur without some kind of coronial enquiry carried out by a local J.P., and this applied even in the Palmer rush except perhaps early in the year of 1874. Thousands of Chinese were off loaded at Cooktown and a certain number of these disappeared on the road to the diggings without trace. (In 1879 there were 15000 Chinese in a total population of 15800 on the Palmer River.) By 1875 however, social order had once again been established. This was true of all North Queensland. In 1866, for example, Governor Bowen could communicate with Landsborough on the Albert River in the Gulf; and telegraph lines rapidly followed settlement even if roads did not.

I have studied the population at risk and deaths for the year 1875 combining the Palmer River and Cooktown districts.[131] The crude death rate was 19–20 per 1000 of population. The crude death rate for the whole of the state for 1875 was 23.8/1000. However, of the deaths used to calculate the latter, at least 40% would have been in young children of whom there were very few in these two northern districts. Hence, 19–20/1000 is high by the standards of the time for a population of males of working age. How high it is difficult to say — probably about twice or three times as high as might have been expected. The crude death rate among civilians of military age in the United Kingdom, for the period 1817–36, was 11.5.

As it happens, there was another working group in Queensland who also were mainly adult males in the prime of life. These were the Kanakas. Thus, it is legitimate to compare the death rates . The Kanakas' crude death rate in 1875 was 85 per 1000, and most of these occurred in southern Queensland. The Palmer by comparison was salubrious! It is a paradox that the adult group with the highest death rates recorded in colonial Queensland were the dark skinned Kanakas, the Melanesians introduced to do the labouring work. We gave them our diseases.

It should be remembered also that elsewhere in the colony there were from time to time fever outbreaks which produced quite high fatality rates. One such occurred among workers and their families building the Dalby–Roma railway line. The patients overwhelmed the Toowoomba Hospital, overflowed into Ipswich and Brisbane, and actually were lodged even further afield than this at Peel Island. This epidemic was officially investigated by Bancroft. The fever probably was malaria, but it may well have been typhoid.[132]

We must also keep a sense of proportion. Derrick[133] has demonstrated in a graph that the highest number of deaths recorded as due to typhoid in North Queensland occurred in the 1880s. At the worst these numbered about 100 per annum. This can be translated into a death rate of about 160/100000 of general population (North Queensland). In 1885 the death rate from typhoid for the whole colony was 85/100000 but it had been as high as 185/100000 in 1883. (The case fatality rate for typhoid in Brisbane ranged from 8% to 12%).[134] Some 2% became 'carriers' of the disease. They contrived to pass the bacteria in their faeces and caused further outbreaks of the disease. The bacteria attack the walls of the small intestine and may cause the walls to perforate. At the time of writing the male death rate from ischaemic heart disease in Australia is 307/100000.[135] Is this holding up the development of Australia and deterring migration?

Malaria, however, was the crucial disease. If malaria had had a different natural history in Queensland the settlement of the north may not have been so felicitous. What, for example, would have been the course of our history if the area had been hyperendemic with a high proportion of malignant malaria? Breinl in his Stewart lecture remarked that Cairns —

...was at times a hot bed of virulent malaria. 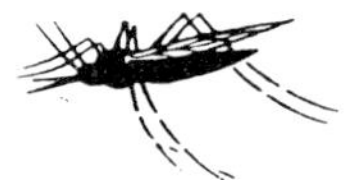

The local authority part-time Medical Officer, Baxter Tyrie, refuted this and was not contradicted when he claimed that, irrespective of what happened years ago, the residents of Cairns had in recent times enjoyed a healthy environment. He aggrievedly pointed out that such unfounded and sweeping statements would adversely affect the tourist trade!

Both Ford[136] and Black[137] have discussed the problem of malaria in Australia. Over most of the endemic area, that is, in the Gulf and Peninsula, the population has been sparse and tended to be static except for bursts of mining activity. The vector in the Peninsula is seasonal and in some seasons may not occur at all. Furthermore, malignant malaria is relatively uncommon and when it has appeared it has always been after a recent introduction to Queensland. In those areas on the eastern coast, particularly around Cairns, the economic and social infrastructure has been sufficient to make control effective. Our 'triumph in the tropics' has been aided by a fair element of good fortune bestowed by natural conditions. (*See Endnote 4*)

Derrick[138] took the view that the present position in respect to malaria is "an uneasy and qualified victory". In my opinion, as long as the economy of these areas remains sound there is little likelihood that malaria would ever become a serious menace, though there might be localized outbreaks from time to time, as has occurred in Cairns and Torres Strait. In this I put my faith primarily in dollars and the general education that results therefrom, rather than in doctors.

Summary of "dysentery and fevers"

Dysentery and typhoid can be prevented by good hygiene, and this is what gradually happened. Even small technical advances helped. Landsborough wrote in 1866[139] about using "zinc coated iron sheets", galvanized iron, at Sweer's Island. In old photos of early North Queensland homes, it can be seen that a number have gutterings and tanks. Hence, apparently such materials were available fairly early in our colonial history. Square iron tanks ('ships' tanks) were still common water receptacles in my youth around country homesteads. At least the drinking water came from rain water collected in a tank even if water for ablutions, gardens etc. was drawn from a communal water hole or stagnant creek. 'Ships tanks' were the mini containers of the 19th century. Tea and other valuable goods were sent to Australia in them.

Even the incidence of malaria is to some extent connected with standards of living. This is seldom appreciated. Gunther[140] recently referred to the decrease in its incidence with the growth of social improvement and stressed a quotation —

Malaria flees before the plough.

Cilento and Baldwin (1930)[141] writing perceptively at an earlier period said the same thing in a different way —

The poor are malarious and the malarious are poor.

Thus we may conclude that the group of diseases — "fever and dysentery" — most liable to cause massive and serious morbidity and mortality, though in isolated incidents alarming, was over all not exceptionally grave for the times.

Hookworm *(See Endnote 5)*

In 1893 the President of the North Queensland Medical Society pointed out that there was evidence to support the supposition that hookworm was present in the north[142] and in the early years of this century the rather alarming incidence of this disease in North Queensland was receiving quite a deal of attention. R. O'Brien[143] who had been full-time medical officer of health under Ham, subsequently settled in practice at Cairns. He was the first medical man to take a microscope to those parts. His early papers drew attention to the hookworm problem. (In one street in Cairns, which was called derisively "Ancylostoma Alley", everyone was said to have the disease. In a survey in later years, 25% of people in the Cairns shire were found to have the complaint.)[144]

It must be realized, however, that North Queensland settlement had been in existence for 30 years before any concern was expressed about hookworm, and some 50 years before any remedial action of any consequence was taken. As we shall see in Part IV of this paper, the action consisted of a number of specific surveys and campaigns, including a very sophisticated campaign conducted under the aegis of the International Health Board of the Rockefeller Foundation, 1919–1924.

In the five year period (1919–24) 248721 people were examined and 48256 were found to be infested. Most of the patients were in the wet tropics with, in addition, an enclave of sufferers around Nambour (high rainfall area), in all coal mines (defaecation underground in warm moist conditions) and in mental disease institutions. From 1922 onwards the survey included a search for malaria and filariasis, but few 'positives' were discovered.[145]

All eventually agreed that hookworm infestation was the only tropical disease of any numerical importance in North Queensland. (Approximately 20% of the population examined was infested. In children 6–18 years the percentage = 40%.) But what of its effects? Waite and Nielsen considered that the disease retarded development in children — physically and mentally. (In 1919 they published alarming pictures which showed pairs of children of the same age; in each pair one child had hookworm, the other was free from it; the latter child, in each case, was much bigger than the other. They published, as well, graphs showing "I.Qs" of children; those with hookworm had lower "I.Qs".)[146]

But earlier than this, J.S.C. Elkington[147] in his annual report for the year ending 30th June 1911, had written of hookworm as follows:

> *This disease does not appear so far to have wrought any serious, permanent or racial damage in Queensland, and extensive personal observation on children in many northern localities has failed to show evidence of physical or moral deterioration of the kind recorded by Stiles, Dock and other American observers in certain of the Southern States.*

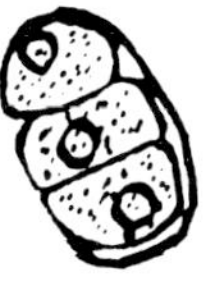

What was the truth? In the final report of the Australian Hookworm Campaign (1924), the summing up seemed to support Elkington.[148]

There was no doubt that from time to time, some individuals died of hookworm infestation — either directly or indirectly;[149,150,151] but in the main, if the child's diet was good, development was not greatly affected and in adult life the parasites were gradually lost. Those most likely to be adversely affected were aborigines who had the maximum rate of infection, the maximum parasite load and the poorest diet. This conclusion would, in the main, coincide with modern views on the subject. Unless malnutrition and/or chronic anaemia from some other cause, such as malaria, are present, the effects of hookworm infestation are not likely to be serious.

The Director-General of Health and Medical Services (Q) in his Annual Report for 1968–69 noted that of 598 faecal specimens which had been examined in North Queensland, none had been positive for hookworm.[152]

Once again we were dealing with a filth disease. It was simply a matter of building sound lavatories and persuading the population to use them.

Ophthalmia

This disease occurred all over Australia in the 19th century. In Queensland, ophthalmia was not restricted to the tropics but was a common problem throughout our settlements commencing with the Moreton Bay convict days.[153] It is essentially a disease associated with poor hygiene and crude conditions of living. May (1958)[154] stated:

> *The civilization of a people can be assessed by the number*
> *of its trachoma patients.*

And again:

> *Trachoma recedes before the advance of civilization ...*
> *Its incidence is in direct relation to social rank.*

After World War I its incidence tended to be confined to western areas of Queensland, but even in the years immediately after World War II the State Health Department still found it necessary to send an ophthalmologist on an annual tour of the schools in the far west of the State. Between the Wars there was a special hospital/hostel in

Brisbane to treat children suffering from the complaint. Ophthalmia, however, is not the kind of disease which would have held up settlement, particularly among males, since only a few who had the affliction suffered serious consequences. Most of our ophthalmia was not true trachoma. (*See Endnote 6*)

It is one of the 'filth' diseases. Finger contact, flies, and even the use of roller towels in schools all have been implicated. Where water was scarce and personal washing facilities deficient, ophthalmia was prevalent, often in epidemics. When North Queensland was being settled it was particularly common in the dry areas of western Queensland.

Alcoholism

This, of course, is a common problem rendered worse in pioneering communities where there is a great excess of males, few social diversions and little control over the numerous outlets which sell 'grog' of dubious quality. It is hardly a disease which is confined to tropical areas. Most medical experts in the north would have agreed with Hunt's statement (1892):[155]

There is, however, an enormous amount of preventable disease for which alcoholic excess is largely responsible.

An editorial comment in 1910[156] remarked that alcohol rather than cane cutting put a strain on North Queensland workers. This was quoting Breinl.

There is not the slightest doubt that alcoholism in tropical Australia has caused greater problems than any so called tropical disease.

Skin disease

Diseases affecting the skin had a relatively high incidence. The northern European in tropical Queensland had twice the chance of developing skin cancer as he had at the latitude of Brisbane.[156a,b,c] And there was as well an increased incidence of common skin conditions.[157, 158, 159, 160] Pterygia also in North Queensland occur readily.

None of these conditions, however, were particularly life threatening. and in many cases they hardly constituted even a nuisance. Today, man's skin, which he exposes directly to the insult of a tropical climate, presents the only disease entities of numerical consequence which still affect Queenslanders as a result of living in the northern parts of the state. Pterygia, skin cancers and 'dermatitis' are common.

Other disease entities

Diet

Not surprisingly there were deficiencies of diet. In the dry western areas 'Barcoo rot' (an indolent sore) and 'Barcoo spew' were not uncommon. They probably were due to a dietary deficiency, but were not of sufficient import to hold up settlement.

'Sprue' was seen in patients on the coast from time to time, but numerically was not of importance.

Beri Beri

This was noted particularly among pearling crews at Thursday Island. I found the following also in the *Brisbane Courier* suggesting that the Chinese on the Palmer River goldfield were suffering from Vitamin B deficiency:

> *... 25 Chinese in Cooktown Hospital with paralysis of the lower extremities*[161]

and, again in the same paper:

> *... 70 patients in Cooktown Hospital, 45 of whom are Chinese, nearly all affected with paralysis, the usual and only complaint perennial here, caused by over-loading themselves as packers to the Palmer. Cooktown is remarkably healthy ...* [162, 163]

Plague

The effects of plague were experienced mainly from 1900 to 1908, but these were much more disruptive in Brisbane than in North Queensland. Cumpston and McCallum[164] state that in the relevant period (1900 to 1908) there were 102 patients suffering from plague in North Queensland and 51 of these died.

Filariasis

This disease was said to have been introduced by the Kanakas and was present in North Queensland. However, its incidence was higher in southern Queensland. At one stage in Brisbane, 10 to 17 per cent of people examined had filarial parasites in their blood.[165, 166, 167]

Leprosy

This was reputed to have been introduced by the Chinese coming to the goldfields. Patients suffering from the disease were found from time to time all over the state, but the numbers were not large. For reviews, see Thompson[168] and Cook.[169]

And thus we come to an end of our consideration of those specific diseases in the causation of which tropical living may have played a major part. It is not surprising that the popular literature of the time and various 19th century biographies which have come down to us showed no major concerns with problems of health.

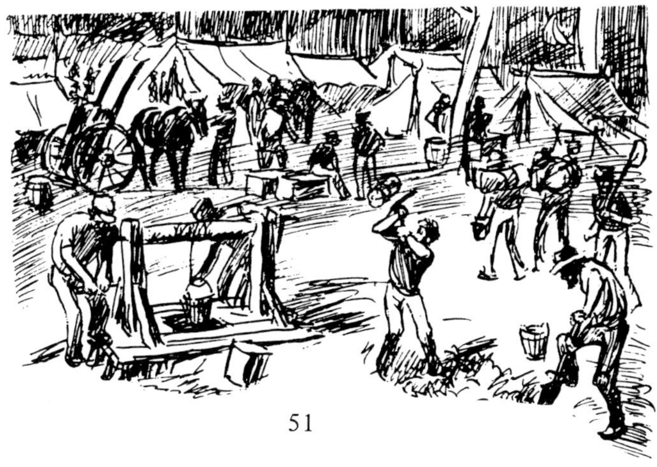

THE EFFECTS OF CLIMATIC STRESS

The effect of tropical climatic stress is a threat rather different from that posed by tropical disease. It is seen as a factor which produces very long term results and, as a consequence, members of a group of European migrants would fail as the generations go by to perpetuate their genes and their culture. They would die out.

Almost crucial to the doctrine of climatic determinism was the belief that settlement in North Queensland must inevitably sooner or later be disastrous for northern Europeans, due to stresses imposed by the climate.

This was well stated by Nisbet[170] pere (Townsville), one of the few doctors who actually worked in North Queensland, whom I can find recorded as being pessimistic about northern settlement. At the 1911 Intercolonial Medical Congress he said :

> *... our race is dwindling away to a few highly exotic anaemic people incapable of producing their species, unless fed with a constant strain of European immigration.*

He went on to say that the women had mammary development too deficient to sustain child rearing, that they were infertile and that their children were over given to convulsive seizures.

The other northern practitioners did not agree that this was a statement of present fact; but as a long term prediction, no one was quite sure whether he was right or wrong.[171, 172, 173, 174] So much was this so that the Congress passed a resolution urging the Commonwealth Government to support the Australian Institute of Tropical Medicine more generously, and made the health of people living in tropical Australia the plenary topic for the Australian Medical Congress to be held in Brisbane in 1917. But War intervened and that Congress was not held until 1920.[175]

Atlee Hunt much later summed up this controversy succinctly :

> *... it was freely alleged on the one hand that it was physically impossible for white people to perform hard work in the tropics and maintain their health, and on*

the other, that the question was not one of health or climate, and that though certain inconveniences and discomfort were no doubt inseparable from life in hot countries there were no reasons on the ground of health to prevent white people from performing manual work in the Australian tropics.[176]

By 1920 Breinl was able to give his views, based on ten years of investigation in North Queensland.[177, 178, 179] This could be summarized in terms of evidence given by him to the Queensland Industrial Court and Industrial Commission in 1921. This ran along the following lines:

(1) the absence of any worthwhile incidence of tropical diseases (hookworm excepted)

(2) a climate which per se posed no real threats to health

(3) a climate which, on really hot days, caused marked discomfort and thus a climate in which mental activity sometimes required some degree of determination. (Macpherson (1949)[180] has pointed out that a tropical climate can be trying and aggressive.)

There was also presented at the 1920 Congress actuarial evidence which did not suggest any excessive mortality in North Queensland.[181] The result was that, in the main, members of Congress were inclined to think that the stresses of living in Northern Australia were mainly psychological. A letter from P.A. Mapleston[182] once a staff member of the Institute, and the report of the 1920 Congress also sum up the final conclusions very well.[183]

The opinion in the ensuing fifty years has not altered greatly. When the Medical Faculty commenced in Queensland (1936), its School of Physiology under D.H.K. Lee, who himself had come originally from North Queensland, constituted as its major research activity, an investigation into human adaptation to hot climates. Lee and his associates introduced to Australia the concept and methods of assessing climatic stress accurately; and, as a result, they were able to define more precisely the various regional climates in Queensland. Perhaps more importantly, they were able to show the practical applications of their findings to house design, to ventilation and to cooling. This has had quite a marked effect in the field of architecture and ventilation. Lee's attitude to air conditioning in hot climates should be mentioned. Among Australians he was a precursor in realizing that it was as logical to cool the environment in the tropics as to heat it in a cold climate.

Breinl and his associates raised the question of urinary concentration in hot climates and its possible influence as a factor in causing chronic renal tract disease, without coming to any definite conclusions. More recent work has shown that cane cutters suffer water and salt depletion by the end of the day.[184] Then, after Breinl, nephritis and the 'lead story' occupied Queensland medicine for many years. However, at the present time, for reasons which still are largely unknown, there does seem to be an excess mortality from renal tract disease in this state.[185] Whether or not North Queensland shows a higher incidence than the southern parts of the state, I do not know.

One subsequent investigation was definitive. This was carried out under the direction of Patrick.[186] He showed that children who had lived all their lives in the tropics and whose parents had lived all their lives there, were in no way inferior to their southern counterparts.

Dam, a psychologist, has done much the same in respect to performance in school.

These investigations were important because they gave a precise answer to that often propounded bogey of racial degeneration. Children had been examined before, but somewhat earlier in the century before the alleged detrimental factors may have had time to do their worst!

Ellesworth Huntington[187] at the end of a long professional life, was confounded by events which the passage of time had brought about and by the experiences of World War II, but he was not converted. He could still protest and prophesy gloom. He commented thus about life in a hot climate:

> *Leisurely rest and social amenities get more time than in more bracing climates, whereas such matters as serious reading, inventions, new projects and the promotion of education, health and good government got less. Activity of this latter type are by no means absent, but they proceed more slowly than among people of similar ability, character and training in more stimulating climates.*

There the story rests. The present vigour of various North Queensland industries and the enthusiasm with which its citizens promote these industries, their communities and their university undertaking at Townsville, supply little support for Huntington's gloomy prediction.

The strange paradox about the whole story is this. Pessimism has seldom come from people actually living in the North; the tragic chorus has nearly always been supplied by those who live in temperate climates.

The history of ill health in the last half of the 19th century in Australia was dominated by tuberculosis, typhoid and deaths in children under five years of age. The discovery of gold in 1851 exacerbated all social and health problems. In one decade the population of Australia increased at least 2½ times, whereas it took about four decades after World War II for the Australian population to double.

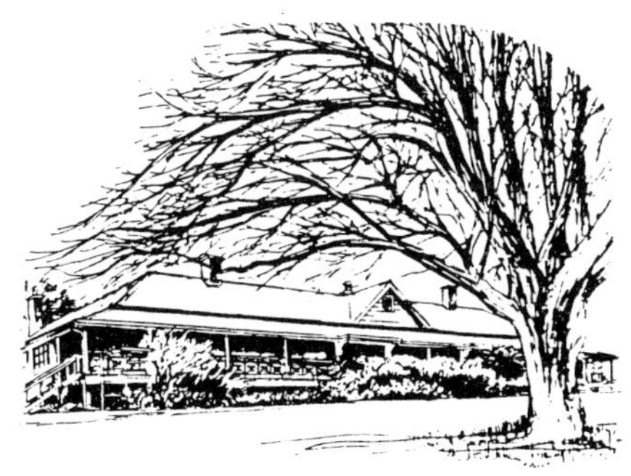

Tropical Australia affords a unique opportunity for studying the adaptability of the white race to a tropical climate and conditions, not only of a white race surrounded by a host of native servants, but of a white race doing hard manual labour under a tropical sun. Results obtained in this direction would be of great economic importance, not only for Australia but for the tropics in general.

(From Breinl's first report 1910, quoted by Cilento and Lack in "Triumph in the Tropics", p. 435, 1959, Brisbane, for the Historical Committee of the Centenary Celebrations Council of Queensland)

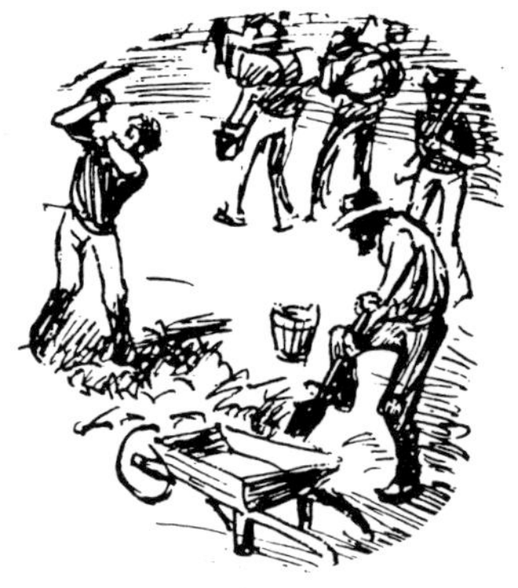

PART IV

MEETING THE CHALLENGE

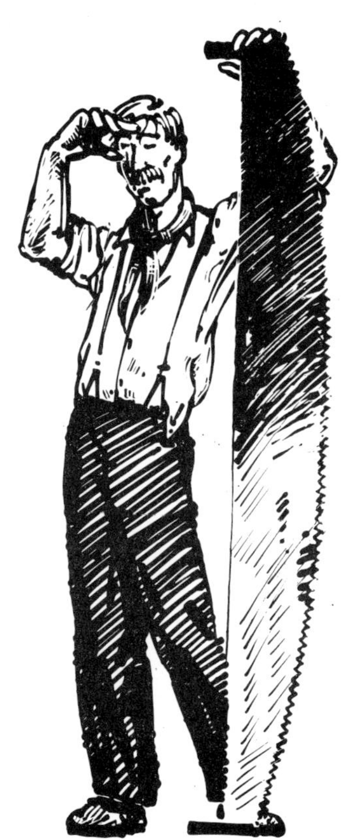

ery little of a specific nature was done to prevent disease in tropical Queensland until after the turn of the century. However, hospitals were established in most centres of any size and eventually most of the towns in which they were sited became connected by rail. (Thursday Island, Cooktown and Mossman were obvious exceptions.) As mentioned already, viable industries gradually produced a healthier environment.

In this part I will discuss:

- Public Health Administration in North Queensland, and

- Measures taken to prevent disease.

When some interest in public health, (the preventive measures which a community carries out as a collective body), was evinced around the turn of the century, then it was because of several factors:

1. The controversies which had enmeshed health in North Queensland with the "White Australia" policy, the departure of the Kanakas and the price of sugar.

2. The advent of plague in 1900, mainly in southern Queensland. (This led to the appointment of a Public Health Commissioner. This was the first occasion in which there was a medical practitioner with a full time vested interest in public health in the state (or colony)).

3. The environmental sanitation movement of the last half of the 19th century had captured the interest of sundry reformers and members of the medical profession. *(See Endnote 7)*

The medical profession demonstrated this quickened interest in public health by discussions at the various medical congresses from that of the Fifth Session at Brisbane in 1899 (Intercolonial Medical Congress) to the Eleventh Session, back again to Brisbane in 1920 — now the Australasian Medical Congress.[188, 189, 190, 191]

The actual practice of public health, however, had to become the responsibility of governments, both the Federal Government and the State Government of Queensland. It is the somewhat unusual form which this public health administration took which will now be discussed.

PUBLIC HEALTH ADMINISTRATION

Centralization

In the last half of the 19th century in the United Kingdom the newly devised practice of public health had been entrusted to 'boards of health' set up by the local authorities. The government instituted a central board of health acting more or less in an advisory capacity. (In my view this was really making a virtue of necessity; it was impossible to impose any real power over the intense parochialism found among local authorities in the United Kingdom.)

This system had been copied in the colony of Queensland, but had little or no effect because in most cases members of local authorities had no interest in promoting good health. The Joint Board of Health, for example, which was supposed to carry out the responsibilities of preventing disease on behalf of local authorities in the metropolitan region, was, judging by its works and its conduct, one of those institutions destined to turn sour all men and matters which it touched.

When Ham was appointed as first Commissioner of Public Health on 1st January, 1901[192, 193] he took over the somewhat vague powers of the Central Board which was abolished. Then all local health boards were abolished in 1902.

Responsibility for preventing plague was removed altogether from the local authorities and this power was not restored to them until 1916.[194, 195, 196, 197]

The conduct of some local boards was almost unbelievable. The Joint Board in Brisbane, for instance, would not furnish Ham with the names of plague patients admitted to the Colmslie Quarantine Hospital. At one stage it tried the ploy of saying that the epidemic probably was not plague. On another occasion it suggested that their nuisance inspector (an untrained man) knew more about the matter than Ham, who had a postgraduate diploma in public health.[198, 199]

Australia as a whole had rendered lip service mainly to the 'health board' system and has not committed major authority in public health administration to local authorities. But this process of centralizing power in state health departments certainly displayed its most florid manifestations in Queensland.

In my opinion this was almost of necessity due to the antagonistic attitudes to public health practice shown by most members of local authorities. Hence the responsibility for public health practice in tropical Queensland tended to be controlled from Brisbane.

Non-graduate field staff

In two other states at least public health activities in regions outside the metropolitan area were entrusted to the supervision of medical graduates who were full time experts in that branch of medicine. These were district health officers. We might therefore have expected to find doctors of this kind in North Queensland who were permanent salaried officers of the State Health Department.

In fact, in January, 1913, a full time regional medical officer, Booth Clarkson, had been appointed to Townsville.[200, 201] His successor was King Patrick, the second and last encumbent. This office was deliberately abolished in May, 1916 while Dr Patrick was still there, not because there was difficulty in obtaining staff, but because it was considered unnecessary to retain full time medical officers outside Brisbane. [202, 203] The State Health Department provided medical control from Brisbane.

The local authorities depended for public health advice on part time medical officers who were clinicians with practices in the vicinity. Their emolument was paltry and the amount of time they devoted to public health was usually in proportion.

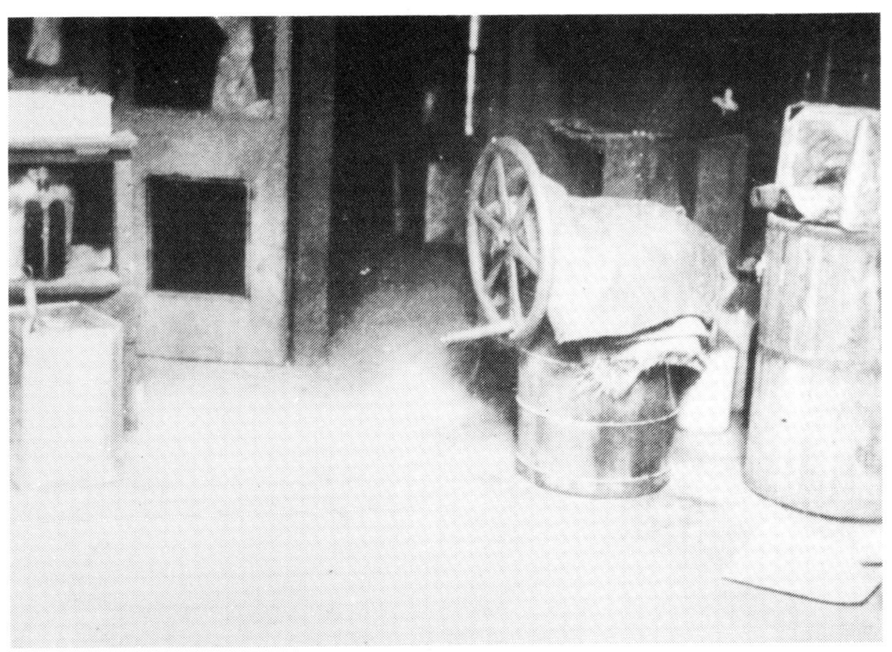

Health inspectors played a very significant role in improving the standards of hygiene in North Queensland.
This photograph shows an early ice-cream factory in a northern town.

The State Health Department delegated its responsibilities outside Brisbane to health inspectors and nurses and not to medical officers.

Today in developing countries it is advocated that promotion of health in villages and in other field situations should be left to non-graduates. This is considered very innovative. Queensland used this system successfully sixty to seventy years ago.

This Queensland exercise in 'doing it without doctors' did not seem to bring down the thunderbolts of the gods. For quite a number of years in this century while all this was going on, this state had the lowest infant mortality rate (outside New Zealand) in the world. (Actually the connection between the number of doctors in a community and its infant mortality rate is a complex matter.)

Specialist Units

The other peculiar feature of Queensland Public Health administration was the tendency to set up specific units to handle specific disease problems. For example, there was a Weil's Disease Inspectorate to control leptospirosis in sugar cane fields, a hookworm inspectorate to maintain surveillance in that disease and a medical officer, (an ophthalmologist), originally within the Department of Public Instruction, travelled around the west of the state to control ophthalmia.

There was also a trend to set up special investigations carried out by organizations outside the control of the State Health Department. The most remarkable of these was the Australian Institute of Tropical Medicine set up at Townsville in 1910. In more recent years the Queensland Institute of Medical Research conducted a field station at Innisfail to study 'coastal fevers'. During World War II the Army contributed something to the study of malaria and scrub typhus, and more recently the Queensland University (Department of Social and Preventive Medicine) studied the incidence and prevalence of skin cancers.

The Hospitals

The social and economic development of North Queensland was such that most who were seriously ill ended up in a hospital of some kind. This may not have applied immediately after the opening up of the country, but certainly not long after. For instance, there was a well established hospital at Cooktown during the Palmer River gold rush. This has meant that it was hardly likely that any serious disease problem would go unnoticed.

The hospitals served as a centre for unofficial study of local patterns of disease and many of the doctors had leisure and were keen observers. Some went to small outback hospitals where the work was not particularly demanding because of chronic ill health. I personally have known two of these — E.H. Derrick, with tuberculosis, who spent a number of years in North Queensland's small towns, and Mervyn Patterson, who went to Aramac because of severe cardio-spasm. In different ways, both subsequently contributed to preventive medicine — one in research and the other as a distinguished part time medical officer of health who introduced diphtheria immunization to this state.

I will devote the rest of this part to describing specific undertakings which have contributed to an improvement in health in tropical Queensland.

SPECIFIC INVESTIGATIONS AND MEASURES OF PREVENTION

David Hardie (1893)

Dr Hardie correlated local meteorological details with disease incidence, helped by the Colonial Statistician and the Colonial Meteorologist. Hardie was a well known Brisbane physician and very definitely part of the 'establishment'. This produced very little of practical value.[204]

Australian Institute of Tropical Medicine (A.I.T.M.) 1910

I will treat of this at some length later.

Hookworm survey and surveillance

1. Preliminary survey undertaken by the Queensland Government aided by the Australian Institute of Tropical Medicine. (Elkington, who became Commissioner of Public Health (after Ham) in 1910, was very interested in problems of tropical health.)

2. In 1916 the Federal Government persuaded the International Health Board of the Rockefeller Foundation to help Australia assess its hookworm problem. (Elkington had gone over to the Federal Quarantine Service in 1913.) He became the Director of its Division of Tropical Hygiene based in Brisbane. No doubt he now influenced both governments — state and federal.[205]

   A preliminary survey was carried out in New Guinea followed by a pilot survey in North Queensland under the direction of an American, J.H. Waite,[206, 207] and later S.R. Lambert.[208] The A.I.T.M. assisted with this.

3. The five year survey. This was carried out from 1st October 1919 to 30th September 1924 by "The Australian Hookworm Campaign". Budget: £100,000, expenditure £93,784. Federal Government contributed 35%, Queensland, 28.6%, 'Rockefeller', 30%. First W.A. Sawyer and then W.C. Sweet were in charge. All coastal Queensland and the northern rivers of New South Wales were covered.

4. Joint Federal-Queensland Campaign (1925–1932). Initially the Federal Government contributed £4000 per annum, Queensland, £3500 and New South Wales, £500. The Director of Tropical Hygiene Division was an ex officio Director of the Campaign. His deputy was the Director of the A.I.T.M.[209, 210]

5. Hookworm Inspectorate — Queensland Government. This inspectorate has been based on Cairns and has functioned without federal aid since 1932. It does not have a medical director but is supervised by public health doctors based on Brisbane.[211]

Commonwealth Health Laboratories at Townsville and Cairns

The regional Commonwealth Laboratories were established to work in conjunction with large regional public hospitals. They were a federal contribution to assist rural areas which lacked facilities for laboratory investigation of disease. This was to assist clinical practice, that is, treatment of patients. As well as supplying ancillary facilities to clinical practice they acted as 'public health' laboratories. The years of establishment were: Townsville, 1922; Cairns, 1928; Rockhampton, 1924. the facilities offered by these laboratories indirectly helped research.

This was illustrated by an investigation of leptospiroses among cane cutters at Ingham in 1933. Dr Gordon Morrissey of Ingham made the clinical report and the laboratory at Townsville did the serology, assisted by staff from the School of Public Health and

Tropical Medicine in Sydney. Dr Tim Cotter, then at the laboratory in Townsville and later of Innisfail, played a prominent part. As a result, various new leptospiral strains were discovered. This work thus gave an entity to at least one group of fevers occurring in North Queensland.[127, 128, 212]

School of Physiology, University of Queensland

Under the guidance of D.H.K. Lee, a prolonged investigation of tropical fatigue and human adaptation to tropical climates was undertaken from 1936 onwards. Lee and R.K. Macpherson of that school carried out a survey of tropical fatigue in the armed services in the south-west Pacific region during World War II. The practical nature of their work proved of substantial use to the armed services.

Laboratory of Pathology and Microbiology, State Health Department

This laboratory under Derrick's direction in the years prior to World War II discovered the causal micro-organisms for Q fever and Pomona fever in southern Queensland. Shortly after World War II, E.H. Derrick moved on to the Queensland Institute of Medical Research and Dr John Tonge became the laboratory's director. It was then carrying out the serology for northern fevers and with fruitful results. Ten additional serotypes of leptospirae were discovered in North Queensland and five of these had not been described elsewhere in the world. These workers built up a formidable reputation in the zoonoses. In all fifteen leptospiral serotypes have been found in North Queensland and only three of these have been isolated also in southern Queensland. A short paper by Dr J.W. Smith provides a popular summary of this work.[213]

Anthropometric Survey of School Children, 1951

This has been mentioned above. Dr R.P. Patrick of the School Health Service of the State Health Department carried out this survey at Lee's instigation.[214] The survey studied the physical development of children in many parts of Queensland and found no disadvantage from living in North Queensland.[186]

Field Station at Innisfail of the Queensland Institute of Medical Research, 1951–66

By 1950 it would have been true to say that the microbial causes of fever in North Queensland had been for the most part discovered. However, there was difficulty in practice in making use of such knowledge. For example, in 1950–51 Kennedy *et al*[215] stated that there were 147 patients suffering from severe fever in North Queensland for whom no diagnosis was obtained, in spite of repeated serological investigations. The field station was set up to unravel this complexity of fevers still occurring. In the first phase of operations this was done very effectively. In 1954–55 Doherty produced diagnoses for all but five of the patients suffering from fever whom he investigated. In the second phase, the field station carried out a fauna survey; and in its third and last was concerned with arthropod borne viruses.[216] This led to the discovery of Ross River fever and elucidated certain important aspects of Murray Valley Encephalitis. (C.N. Sinnamon had commenced the Field Station.)

Survey of Atypical Mycobacteria

This was conducted by the Chest Clinic Services of the State Health Department in all areas of Queensland but had particular relevance to Central and North Queensland.[217] This demonstrated the relatively high incidence of sub-clinical infections due to atypical mycobacteria in the hotter areas of the state. Sometimes clinical manifestations did occur. E.W. Abrahams was in charge.

Department of Social and Preventive Medicine, University of Queensland

"Regional studies in skin cancer" 1963 and 1966 (Silverstone, Carmichael, Gordon and others). This has been mentioned previously.

Malaria and Scrub Typhus Research

During World War II a study was made of the use of various drugs to suppress the clinical manifestations of malaria. This was carried out by Land Headquarters Malaria Research Unit at Cairns. The successful results had a profound influence on the outcome of military campaigns both in Burma and in the south-west Pacific. At the same time and in the same area the entomological aspects of both malaria and scrub typhus were investigated by the Entomological Research Unit. The work of both these units subsequently received international acclaim. Major Josephine Mackerras (nee Bancroft) was one of the entomologists involved.[218]

These were service investigations not primarily involved with the problems of North Queensland. They were, however, geographically based there.

Destruction of Mosquito Breeding Habitats

At various times and in various places this included extensive drainage programmes.

★　★　★　★　★　★　★

Thus, over a period of almost eighty years the disease problems of North Queensland have been thoroughly investigated within the rather special structure of the state's public health system. Furthermore, two health authorities — state and commonwealth — which at political level go through the motions of much acrimonious dispute from time to time, co-operated very efficiently, as they usually do, in the field and in the market place.

In many ways the North Queensland story has shown how private practitioners, research personnel, public health officials and an allegedly rigid state hospital system can work efficiently and harmoniously in furthering research programmes.

It is of some interest to note that heat stroke and sun stroke have never been problems of any consequence in Australia,[219, 220] though by European standards it was considered a very hot country. Paradoxically, public health authorities often were more concerned about keeping diseases out of tropical Queensland — smallpox, plague, yellow fever, typhus — than they were about those which were there.[221, 222]

Australian Institute of Tropical Medicine

This was Australia's first medical research institute set up to determine the disease load and physiological stress imposed by living in tropical Australia. It was also to give training in tropical medicine and to issue a postgraduate diploma to successful candidates. The diplomas were to be granted by the sponsoring universities and it was envisaged that some of the preliminary academic study might be done in one of the three respective medical schools.[223, 224]

That tropical health problems came to be Australia's first priority in research is a significant indicator of how the White Australia policy and the sugar controversy had impigned on both academic, professional and political interest.

The original instigator had been the Right Reverend George H. Frodsham, Bishop of North Queensland;[225] but it was the three universities with medical schools which set up the Institute and which in theory had the intention of supporting it financially.[226] (Of the initial money Sydney University contributed £150, Melbourne, £100, Adelaide, £50, the Queensland Government £250, and the British Government handed back some money which the Australian Government had been paying to the Imperial Government towards the study of tropical medicine. Knox Darcy of Mt Morgan and Anglo-Petroleum fame gave £1000 for capital costs.)[227]

The Institute came into being in 1910 with an annual income of £600 per annum.[228] The official opening did not take place until 1913.[229] At that function, Anderson Stuart was the only member of the original committee present.[230]

By the time the Report for 1914 was published it carried in small print —

Printed and published for the Government of the Commonwealth of Australia.

The Institute's life as an autonomous academic unit supported by the universities was therefore very brief. There was, in my opinion, nothing surprising or derogatory about this takeover by the federal government. *"He who pays the piper calls the tune"*, and certainly the commonwealth was the most likely source of financial support.

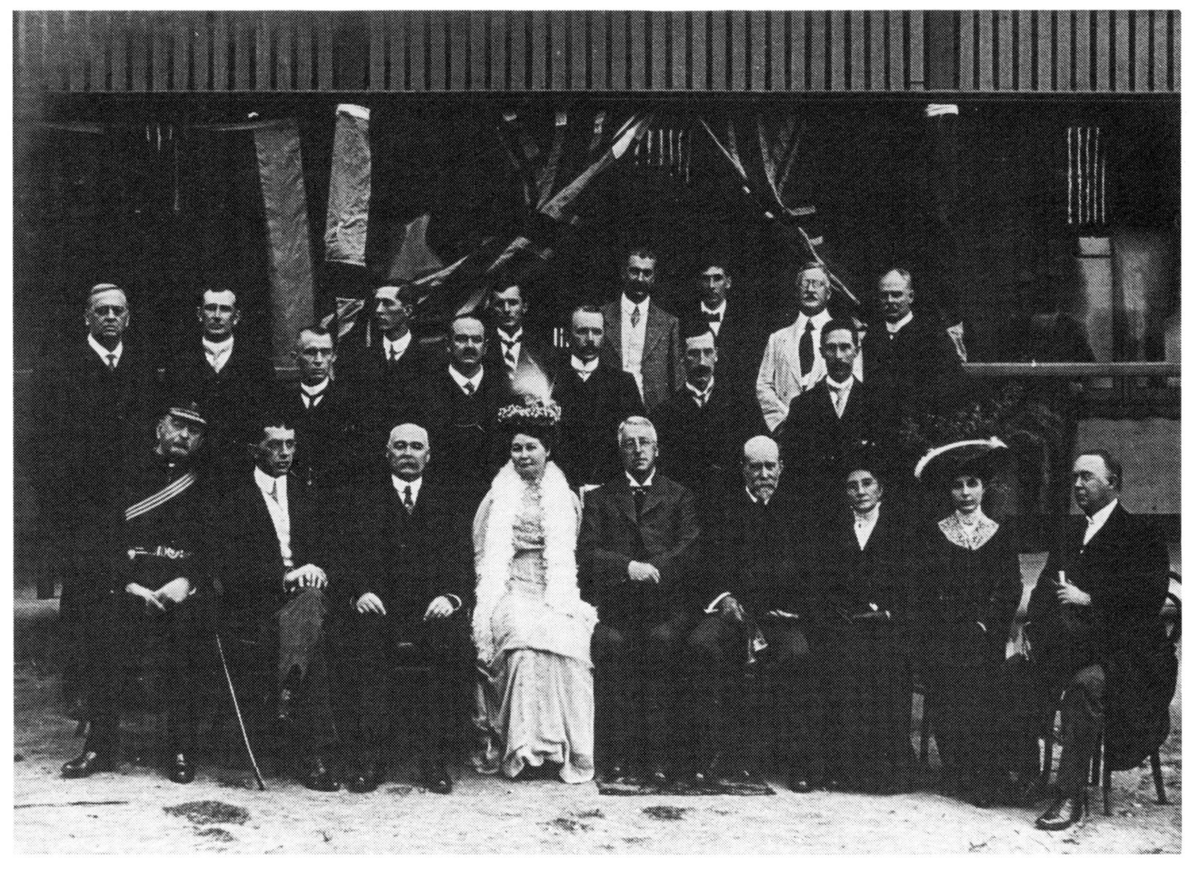

*Opening of the Australian Institute of Tropical Medicine, Townsville, 28th June 1913.
(Photograph by courtesy of The Royal Australasian College of Physicians, Annual Report, 1987)*

BACK ROW *(left to right):*

Mr F.H. Taylor, FRES, Entomologist to A.I.T.M. 1911-1918 and 1925-1945.
Mr J.W. Fielding, FRMS, Laboratory Technician, A.I.T.M. 1910-1954.
Dr C.H. Cormac, Bowen.
Dr W.J. Young, Biochemist to A.I.T.M., 1910-1919.
Dr R.B. Huxtable, Charters Towers.
Dr E. Humphrey, Townsville.

MIDDLE ROW *(left to right):*

Dr C.J. Parkinson, Townsville.
Dr T.G. Ross, Townsville, (Superintendent of the Townsville General Hospital).
Mr Jacob Leu, Townsville (Solicitor), President of the Townsville Hospital Board.
Mr H.C. Johnson, Town Clerk of Townsville.
Captain Foxton, (ADC to Sir William MacGregor).
Dr W. Nicoll, Parasitologist to A.I.T.M., 1912-1915.
Dr H. Priestley, Bacteriologist to the A.I.T.M., 1912-1917.

FRONT ROW *(left to right):*

Dr J Ahearne, Townsville.
Dr A. Breinl, Director, A.I.T.M. 1910-1920.
Mr R.W. McLelland, Mayor of Townsville.
Lady MacGregor, Wife of the Governor of Queensland.
Professor T.P. Anderson Stuart, Professor of Physiology at the University of Sydney, Founder of the
Medical School at that University and one of the founders of the A.I.T.M.
Sir William MacGregor, MD, Governor of Queensland, 1909-1914.
Mrs McLelland, wife of the Mayor of Townsville.
Mrs Anderson Stuart, wife of Professor T.P. Anderson Stuart.
Dr Wilton Love, Brisbane.

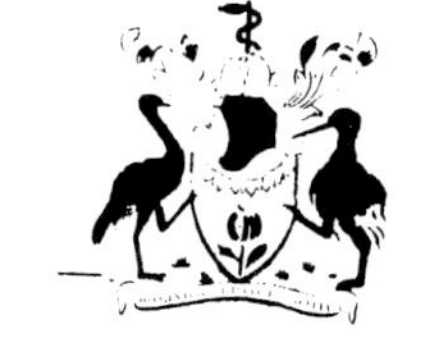

In a moment of initial enthusiastic euphoria the universities no doubt were sincere in their intentions but in reality they had little chance of providing the necessary financial support for the Institute. Medical schools in Australia until very recently have allocated hardly any resources to the teaching of preventive medicine. This occurs because our medical schools have usually been dominated by clinical staff working in large teaching hospitals, an environment in which preventive medicine and public health are not relevant. The exception to this was the Medical School in Queensland which, thanks to Cilento, commenced in 1936 with a somewhat different orientation.

It is no doubt emotionally satisfying to attribute machiavellian intrigue to Cumpston and his federal colleagues, but the reality of the situation was that they had to shoulder a burden which the universities were not prepared to carry.

Breinl, the first director, resigned in 1920[231, 232] and there has been controversy about this ever since. I believe that it occurred because he could no longer stomach the bureaucratic centralized control exercised by Cumpston in Melbourne, and because he wished to raise his income to a level commensurate with his growing family responsibilities. (As an enemy alien during World War I he had experienced some harassment but this was mild compared to that meted out to other medical aliens; and if, as alleged, he had been subjected to really gross derision by his Australian neighbours, it seems strange that he would elect to set up in private practice among them after the War. He also prepared a paper to be read at the Townsville R.S.L.)[233]

To a man such as Breinl, nurtured in the autocracy of Teutonic universities and later in the autonomy of English ones, Cumpston with his inability to delegate and with his obsession about efficiency in administrative detail, would have proved insufferable. Let us hear from P.A. Maplestone, a former staff member. (Maplestone died in July 1969 in Melbourne, full of years and reputation, as one of the best known helminthologists of his generation in the English speaking world.) He wrote the following in 1922:[234]

When I left Australia in July last, the Institute was under the Federal Ministry of Health as a unit of that Department. In addition to controlling from Melbourne the work of the laboratory, the head of this department reserved the right of censorship over all scientific papers written by any member of the staff — a strange state of affairs in an institution whose objects are to determine scientific truths and one not calculated to produce the best results. A second disability was that being part of a large Government department, it had to conform to the routine of that Department — a difficult matter for a research organization, on account of the necessarily irregular nature of the work of the staff. A third objection to the system is that, while no doubt highly capable in their own sphere of governmental methods of administration and the control of public health in a general way, the chief executive officers of such a department have not, nor can they be expected to have, the knowledge or time at their disposal for the direction of a scientific laboratory especially when the laboratory is a long distance away. A first necessity for its future success is the removal of the Institute from the control of the Federal Ministry of Health.

After an interregnum[235] Cilento took charge of the Institute in 1923;[236, 237] but during most of his period in office he was as well supervising Papua–New Guinea's health and medical service. In 1928 he succeeded Elkington as Director of the Division of Tropical Hygiene based in Brisbane. Baldwin was the man on the spot during most of the twenties and often was the Institute's acting director. He conducted the 'long march' south at the end of 1929, and supervised the staff's metamorphosis as part of the School of Public Health and Tropical Medicine (Sydney University) which opened for teaching at the beginning of 1930.

The third controversial point was: Why was the Institute closed and should it have been closed?

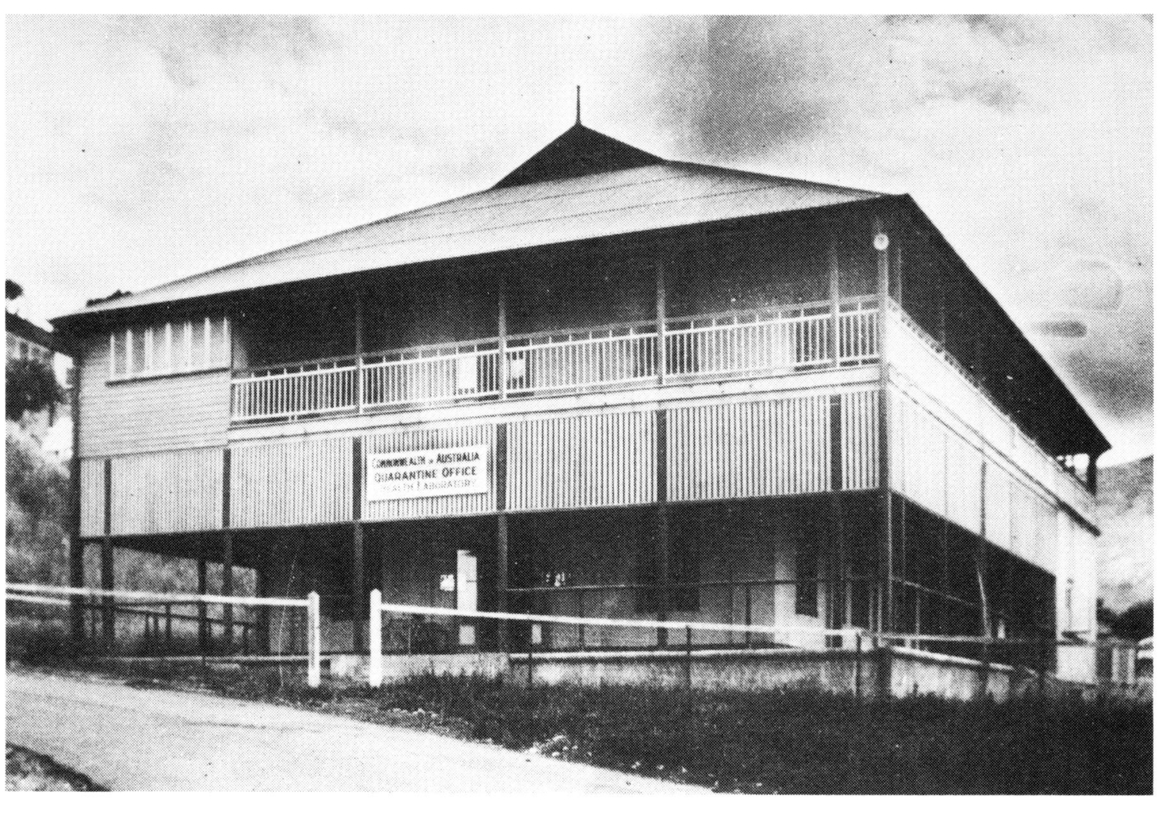

This building housed the Australian Institute of Tropical Medicine, in Townsville.
It provided a focus for the recognition and study of diseases which afflicted both indigenous Aborigines
and caucasian and oriental pioneers in northern Australia. Photograph, courtesy of Fedora Fisher.

In 1933 the Queensland branch of the British Medical Association protested to the federal government about its lack of interest in the health of tropical Australia. Not unreasonably, it pointed out that the Commonwealth Health Department had closed down the A.I.T.M.; had ceased to help the Queensland Government in hookworm control; and had closed down its Division of Tropical Hygiene.[238, 239, 240, 241, 242] My own view is that these withdrawals were due not only to hard times but to a definite change in public health policy.

Given Breinl's report to the Australasian Medical Congress in 1920 and that meeting's findings on the subject, most of the urgency and controversy would seem to have passed from the health problems of living in tropical Australia. That is the first point.

The second point has been made by the 1926 Health Commission.[243] This was the brain child of Hone and Cumpston, and maybe the former was the more perceptive of the two. (One sees Hone's perceptive hand in almost every line of the report.) The Commission and Hone and Cumpston saw the future health problems of Australia as being associated mainly with its cities and their burgeoning industries. Among other things, a centre of excellence for training in public health was badly needed and the A.I.T.M. at Townsville had failed to meet such requirements. Hone and Cumpston faced south and south-east. Elkington and Cilento, on the other hand, were men who faced northwards towards the outer marches of our national domain. They lost, and in my opinion, rightly so. Elkington retired prematurely in 1928, and Cilento resigned from the federal service and became head of the Queensland state health and medical services in 1934.

We can perhaps leave Maplestone to reinforce these views. In this, though hardly a favourite Australian son in Cumpston's eyes — *see above* — nevertheless, in writing the following way back in 1922 he provided reasons for closing the Institute. (Also incidentally it should be noted that the Institute had not been treated badly as far as material resources went; Cumpston was not that kind of ogre.)

The equipment at present there is ample and quite modern enough with which to turn out good work. Many laboratories elsewhere doing valuable work have apparatus no better and often not so good. Moreover, the Institute possesses a scientific library of which it would be difficult to find the equal in any institution of a similar size in the world. It is finding the material of which to employ the apparatus that the difficulties lie. With the possible exception of hookworm disease, which is being dealt with at the present time, none of the tropical diseases mentioned in the article under consideration, nor any of those omitted from it, are causing any hindrance to the settlement of tropical Australia, nor are any of them frequent enough to produce an appreciable economic loss to the country. Research into human disease on a large scale in tropical Australia is an ideal, highly commendable in the abstract, but, like ideals in other walks of life, it may give way before the hard fact that it will not pay.

... and cease for a time at any rate from trying to make poor tropical Australia appear a hot bed of dread diseases for the purpose of trying to stimulate into effectual life a moribund institute.[244]

The cynic will no doubt be intrigued to learn that a decade after Maplestone wrote that, the argument that North Queensland teemed with exotic tropical diseases was used to persuade the state government to establish a medical school in Brisbane — — the right action for the wrong reason!

At all events, there were reasonable arguments for beating a retreat from Townsville in 1930. However, as is so often the case, government authorities failed to appreciate the finer points, the subtleties of life which do so much for morale and which do so much to produce results out of all proportion to the initial outlay. Subsequent events have proved that there was still quite a number of matters of medical interest to investigate in tropical Queensland.

And, apart from what has been done there in the last four decades, (on coastal fevers), which I have already described, a really perceptive mind would have seen the need for a study of aboriginal health. However, since most of us failed to perceive such a need even in the fifties, maybe that is asking too much.

As a matter of interest we are still debating where tropical medicine, now tropical 'health', should be taught. And among other things it is being advocated that the study of tropical disease should be combined with a study of health in deprived ethnic groups such as aborigines, since it has now been realized that the problems arise as much from social and economic factors as from climate.

Before concluding our study of the A.I.T.M. it is necessary to look briefly at its achievements.

Teaching

As well as carrying out research, this institute was to provide instruction for a Diploma in Tropical Medicine, which was to be granted by each of the three universities.[245, 246] It was envisaged that some of the preliminary academic study might be done at the respective medical schools. Two wards at the Townsville Hospital were set aside for use by the Institute's staff. One of these wards was screened. Here clinical experience would be gained; and practical instruction in parasitology would be given in the Institute's laboratory. As it turned out, a deal of bad luck dogged the teaching aspects of activities before World War I; they proved to be quite impossible during the years of that conflict, and were inhibited during the interregnum after Breinl resigned and before Cilento became director. As a consequence, it was not until the last years of the Institute that some diplomas were granted.

I have been able to find records of only four successful diplomates: R.L. Bellamy, 1926; N.B. Watch, 1927; Phyllis Haddow, 1928; C.R. Wiburd, 1928. All were awarded by Sydney University.[247, 248, 249] Sickness had been a problem in the case of some of the candidates.[250] And it was admitted that the Institute did not seem particularly successful in attracting candidates.[251]

Research

On the research side, however, affairs prospered after an initial teething period. Anton Breinl, the first Director, and Fielding, his technical assistant whom he had brought from England, alone were obviously hard put to make up an institute. In 1911 the Ninth Session of the Australasian Medical Congress pressed the federal government for additional financial support. As a result, this was given to the tune of £4000 per annum. The Institute then built up a strong staff. The qualifications of its members were impressive. The research programme was influenced by work being done in the Philippines.[252] The original staff were: Henry Priestley, MB ChM, BSc (Physiology); W. Nicols, MD, DSc, DPH (Parasitology). W.J. Young, MSc, DSc (Biochemistry). Frank Taylor, FES (Entomology); J.W. Fielding (Chief Laboratory Assistant). Nicols and Priestley were termed research assistants and demonstrators.[253]

This team were in the main working on the problems posed by the North Queensland climate in the realm of physiology and disease. The findings were mainly negative. Though this kind of result provided reassurance of local importance in social, economic and political fields, it nevertheless, was not likely to make for great scientific reputations. Valuable prizes are seldom given to those who prove that diseases do not exist. Hence, Breinl's work is largely forgotten. However, I understand that in the fields of general parasitology and entomology quite a number of original findings were recorded. At the beginning of the Institute's activities all was dubiety and obscurity in respect to the effect of the tropical climate. At its end, these doubts had been to a great extent resolved.

What were the achievements? These are recorded in some 150 papers published from the Institute during the twenty years of its existence.[254] Of the people who at various times worked in Townsville, at least six subsequently obtained professorships. These were: Young, Priestley, Maplestone, Baldwin, Lee, Sunstroem and Cilento (part time professorship). A number of others distinguished themselves in other ways in scientific and academic fields. Its research record was certainly meritorious.

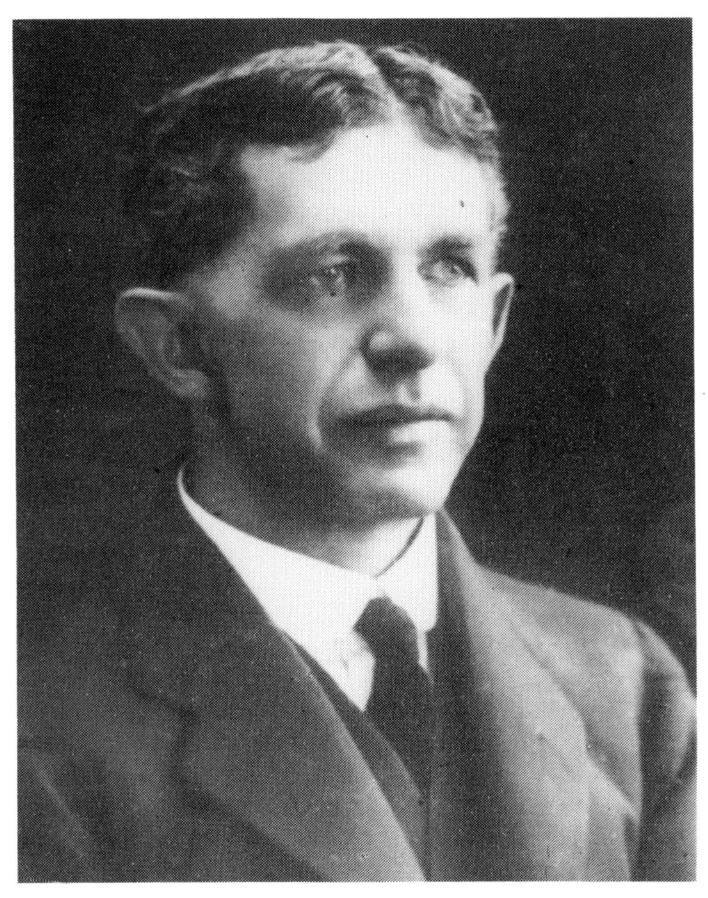

DR ANTON BREINL (1880–1944)

Foundation Director of the Australian Institute of Tropical Medicine, Townsville.

(Dr Robert Douglas, of Townsville, is the acknowledged authority on the life of Dr Breinl)

See: **Douglas RA**. 'Dr Anton Breinl and the Australian Institute of Tropical Medicine', *Med J Aust* 1977; 1: 713-716.
Ibid: 748–751; **Ibid**: 784-790.

Anton Breinl

Finally we must pay a tribute to the Institute's first director. In the first two decades of this century Breinl and Elkington stand out above all others in their grasp of the problems of health in northern Australia. (R. O'Brien after leaving Cairns had a distinguished career, but it was outside Australia.)

Anton Breinl, of Sudeten German origins in Bohemia, was born in Vienna in 1880. He graduated MD in Prague in 1904. The latter city was then part of the Austrian Empire. He became a demonstrator in pathological anatomy with Chiari, came to the Liverpool School of Public Health as the John Garrett International Fellow in Bacteriology; took his Diploma in Tropical Medicine; went on an expedition to Manaos on the Amazon to study yellow fever in 1905; contracted the disease, was invalided home and was shipwrecked on the way.

He was interested in sleeping sickness and in other blood parasites. He was working with a therapeutic substance, atoxyl, an organic arsenical, when he himself became stricken with sleeping sickness due to a laboratory infection. He was the first European to be treated with that drug. This work with atoxyl was a forerunner of Ehrlich's work with arsenicals and was one of the precursors of modern scientific chemotherapeutics.

For the last 2½ years before coming to Queensland, he was Director of the Runcorn Research Laboratories, Liverpool School of Tropical Medicine, to which he had been appointed in 1907. He was basically a protozoologist. C.J. Martin, of the Lister Institute, who was always helpful to the Institute at Townsville and to all Australian medicine, said —

> *In Dr Breinl, the Institute has secured a very strong man*
> *for its first Director.*

He arrived in Townsville in January 1910, a bachelor and recently naturalized. He was at once accorded status as head of Australia's first Institute of Medical Research; his views were frequently quoted in the *Medical Journal of Australia*; he gave the Stewart lectures in 1915, appeared at medical congresses and everywhere seemed to be a highly respected person. He was, as it were, the symbol representing Australian medicine's first rather faltering venture into the glamour world of scientific research.

Shortly after arriving in North Queensland, he was awarded the Mary Kingsley Medal for studies in tropical medicine. Other recipients of the medal at various times were Bruce, Manson, Gorgas, Haffkine, Leonard Rogers, Theobald Smith and Robert Koch. This gives some idea of what the honour meant. He made trips to New Guinea[255, 256] and to the Northern Territory in 1912.[257] During the period that he was at the Institute he investigated at some time or another practically every disease of any importance which cropped up in Northern Australia; and, as well as this, he maintained an abiding interest in the problem of climatic stress. Others were to sort out those North Queensland fevers which at that stage were as yet undefined. Breinl had, however, in his visits to Innisfail and Mossman gone some way towards delineating what these problems were.[258] He realized that, as well as typhoid and malaria, there were at least two others. Thus, he foreshadowed the discovery of scrub typhus and the Australian leptospiroses in North Queensland.

He resigned in October 1920[259, 260] and went into practice in Townsville, particularly interested in general medicine and obstetrics. He was Director of the Institute for almost eleven years. As a clinician Breinl was highly competent and was called upon continually for 'second opinions'. He died in 1944. Though it was twenty-four years since he had actively engaged in research, his obituaries paid tribute to him as one of Australia's most distinguished research workers. I suspect that it was Priestley, a former colleague, who wrote an obituary which said he was —

> *... a splendid man to work with, enthusiastic, very hard working and always ready to give the other fellow more than his share of credit.*

What has impressed me more than anything else in my reading was the manner in which Australia's forgotten scientific man, who had chosen to live in the remote north, was remembered after almost a quarter of a century.

From all accounts given to me by contemporaries, his integrity and other personal qualities matched his scientific talent.[261–266]

SUMMARY

The time has now come to summarize those factors which I believe have favoured successful European settlement in tropical Queensland. And, in conclusion, I must admit that my overall impression is that in the last quarter of the nineteenth century the citizens of North Queensland were worried very little about their health. The major talking point was the Chinese question — "The Yellow Peril" — which they feared was going to overwhelm them. In my opinion the following are the factors which were of importance in aiding successful settlement —

1. The period in the nineteenth century in which northern settlement was started. This was a factor of great importance. In the last half of the nineteenth century the following were available or, subsequent to initial settlement, became available.

   (a) steamship and telegraphic communication which overcame isolation.

   (b) improved technological methods in sugar processing, mining and meat preservation.

   (c) also, the last half of the nineteenth century saw a whole new science developing, namely, knowledge of bacterial and parasitic diseases which in turn made it possible to prevent filth diseases and to discourage urban breeding of certain mosquitoes which were vectors of filariases, dengue and malaria.

   (d) European superiority in weapons and in transport — for example, horses. As a result, aboriginal resistance was destroyed, usually without compunction.

2. A rather fortunate series of circumstances, whereby the three major industries were able to help each other to prosper and to remain economically viable. Furthermore, the presence of the Kanakas provided a form of political blackmail which was to persuade the Australian people of the necessity to financially support a 'white' Australian sugar industry. It also put the industry on its mettle and persuaded the industry to accept orderly marketing. This in turn has led to limitation on the amount of sugar cane which any individual farmer may grow. As a consequence the industry has remained prosperous.

3. A leavening of employers and employees who were superior in experience and initiative to the usual run-of-the-mill European migrant, with a peasant or urban slum background.

4. Migration from and to southern Australia was not impeded by the necessity to obtain passports or work permits.

5. This tropical area benefited from the general social amelioration which was occurring in all western countries. Consequently, better hygiene, improved housing and better diet were as much a product of the times as they were of definite urging from public health authorities.

6. The absence of a numerous indigenous population endowed with a complex social organization which might have resisted the brutal subjugation suffered by the aborigines.

7. By the standard of the times, the 'tropical' disease problems were not particularly gross. They consisted of malaria, 'filth' diseases and certain nutrition

problems of less numerical importance. When eventually there was a will to do something about the two latter, the absence of an indigenous people of alien culture in large numbers made application of the remedies comparatively easy.

Fortunately malaria was not hyper-endemic and it did not require persistent complex measures to break the chain of transmission.[267] The build up of good local hospitals has meant that it is rather unlikely that a large pool of gametocytes — (patients harbouring malaria) — would go undiagnosed and untreated for very long. (In fact, such diagnoses were quickly effected in the outbreak in Torres Strait in 1952.) Even in the late nineteenth century David Hardie had realized that malaria was not a major cause of mortality.[268]

8. (a)   Trade wind tropics with good rainfall and soil suitable for growing sugar cane.

    (b)   Mineral wealth.

In other words, though we must pay our mead of praise to courage, intelligence, resourcefulness and hard work, nevertheless, that intangible ingredient, 'good luck', also played a major part. Its confluence with human endeavour always has moulded history. We might finish with a quotation from Price, who somewhat grudgingly admitted the success of settlement in North Queensland —

If the Australian has done so well by unscientific methods, he will do far better when he adopts scientific plans.[269]

Faced with such an example of condescending patronising airs and graces, maybe the northern paranoia is justified.

ENDNOTE 1

Walter Scott, surgeon, came to Moreton Bay in 1824 and later was prominent in New South Wales. Professor John Pearn has noted that a number of Scott's contemporaries in his home district of Langholm in Scotland became surgeons. Pearn cites six examples of such. All except one would seem to have died when aged thirty or less when serving on various colonial stations. This indicates the dangers of tropical service.[270]

ENDNOTE 2

Some of my social contacts in Victoria even in the 1930s were still bitter about this, particularly since there was a small sugar beet industry in Gippsland. Subsidising a primary industry rankled with many people in other states.

Immediately after federation feelings were even more intense. Any investigation which demonstrated that white labour was incapable of standing up to the physical stress of growing sugar in the tropics would have been welcome. However, that was wishful thinking, since the white miners had already shown that they could carry out hard work in the area. Establishing the Australian Institute of Tropical Medicine at Townsville in 1910, therefore, had popular appeal in circles not ordinarily interested in academic research.

ENDNOTE 3

Throughout the tropical world most indigenous populations had advanced beyond the nomadic stage. They lived in villages and towns. Such people had been the source of so called tropical diseases which threatened the lives of Europeans who had set up outposts in their midst since the 15th century onwards. Native populations transmitted diseases such as malaria, plague, cholera, smallpox, yellow fever etc., both endemically and epidemically. Professor Doherty[271] therefore was perfectly correct in pointing out to me that the nomadic nature of the Aboriginal population made our so called 'triumph in the tropics' relatively easy. Apart from the fact that their social organisation facilitated their subjugation, they were relatively disease free. We tended to give them our diseases rather than the other way around.

However, by the last half of the 19th century, I believe that the presence in tropical Queensland of economically viable industries was the major factor in our success. Filth diseases predominated. A population needs money (from industry) to afford a safe hygienic environment.

The vast areas of the tropics which exist in Western Australia are subject to the North West Monsoon, rather than the Trade Winds. This has made pastoral and agricultural pursuits difficult. Until recently the mining industry was not large. (Now, of course, the area has changed completely due to iron ore, gas, etc.) Living was hard and isolated, though the health of Europeans there probably was as good as at comparable periods in North Queensland. However, the presence of a nomadic population did not protect European populations in Australia from their worst health disaster of all, (apart from the Second and Third Fleets). 'Fever' caused the collapse of the sad little settlements in what is now the Northern Territory, Fort Dundas (1824), Raffles Bay (1827) and Port Essington (1838).

In medical attitudes and knowledge *there was a great difference between the first half and the second half of the 19th century.* To implement this new knowledge required prosperous industry. We also were lucky in respect to communication. Haphazard and irregular contact had been the lot of many colonial outposts in the tropics. This had been disastrous to health. (The only comparable happening in Australia occurred after the landing of the First Fleet.) By the time North Queensland was being settled telegraphic and steamship communication were available all over the area.

My contention is that in the last half of the 19th century medical knowledge had so advanced, especially in respect to sanitation and diseases caused by microbes, that by the time North Queensland came to be settled the health status of the indigenous population was much less important than it had been in past centuries.

Both views are correct. If the indigenous population had been numerous and living in villages and towns when the Europeans first settled in Australia our story, particularly at the present time, would be very different. By contrast, in the last half of the 19th century if money was available for sanitation and education, urban areas in particular in the tropics could be made relatively disease free.

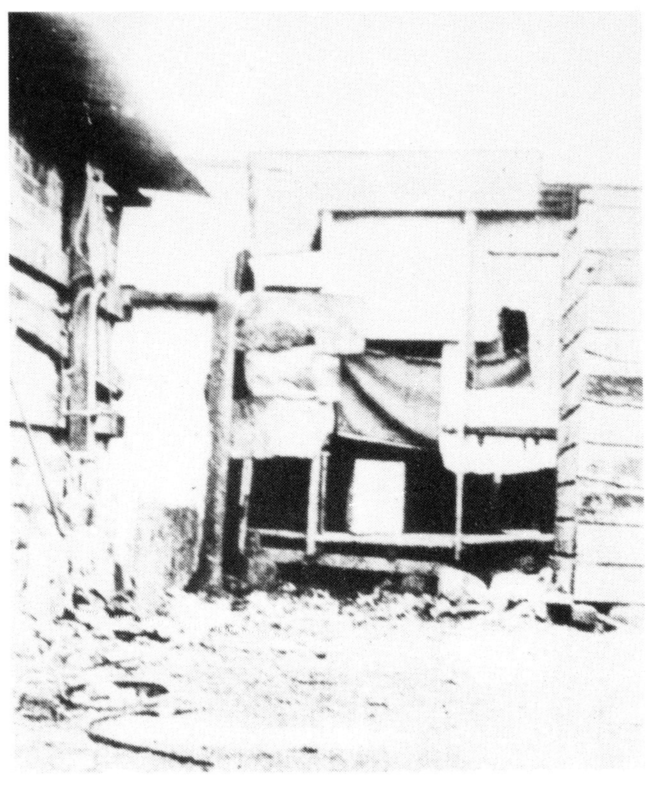

Inadequate sanitation was a major cause of bowel infections
and infestations in the pioneering days
of North Queensland settlement.
This photo shows an earth closet adjacent to a bakery
"in an important northern town", c. 1920.

ENDNOTE 4

Under natural conditions four species of protozoal parasites cause malaria. They all belong to the single genus plasmodium. These parasites are found in the blood stream of human beings who have malaria. They destroy the red cells and, by doing so, cause anaemia.

These parasites are not found in the blood of lower animals. For all practical purposes outside the laboratory the source of infection is another human being. The parasite is transferred from one human to another by the bite of a female anopheline mosquito. However, the species of anopheline varies from place to place in different parts of the world. In North Queensland it is *A farauti.* The parasites undergo a complex life cycle in the gut and salivary glands of the vector mosquito and in the blood stream of the human patient. The blood harbouring parasites in a human population available for transfer by anopheline mosquitoes is called the gametocyte pool.

Of the four protozoal parasites which cause malaria three are regarded as 'benign'. These latter cause prostating acute bouts of fever but seldom cause death unless other diseases such as pneumonia or malnutrition are present. For obvious reasons the presence of malaria in a military campaign can be disastrous, even though most patients do not die. Not only is a patient incapacitated, but extensive medical services are required to look after the victim.

The fourth parasite, *P. falciparum*, behaves very differently. It is termed malignant malaria. Frequently there is brain involvement. If so the outlook is very grave. Fortunately for the settlement of North Queensland this parasite has never persisted in the blood stream of patients. It has caused small isolated lethal outbreaks and has then disappeared until introduced from some source outside Australia, particularly New Guinea.

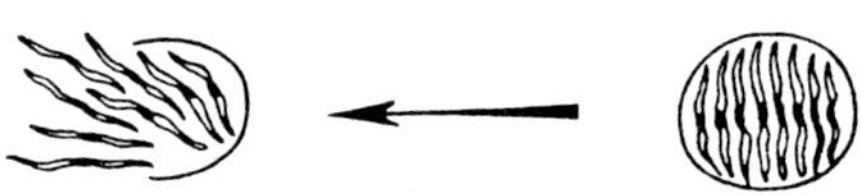

From time to time isolated outbreaks of malignant malaria occurred down the Queensland coast within the range of *A. farauti*, in the Gulf, on the Peninsula and Torres Strait. (*See Fig. 2*) Fortunately a gametocyte pool of *P. falciparum* did not persist.

In cold climates where people may neglect bathing and changing clothes, classical typhus is caused by lice. This disease wrought havoc on convict and migrant ships, but for all practical purposes was never established in Australia. Scrub typhus (mites), tick typhus and murine typhus (associated with grain) occurred in North Queensland and could not be distinguished from malaria, typhoid and leptospirosis.

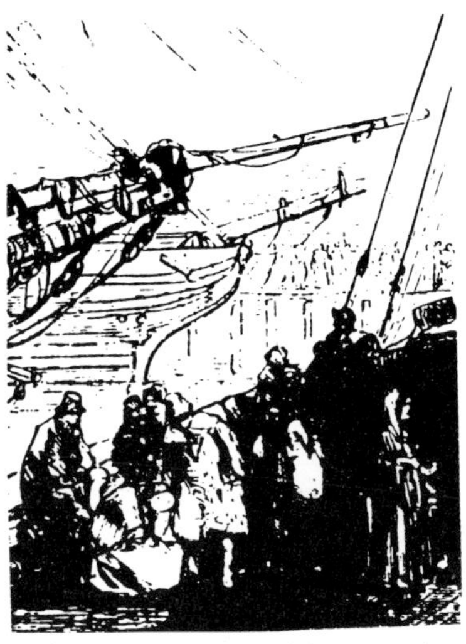

ENDNOTE 5

Hookworm

This disease is caused by a small round worm. Its host is human. A person with the disease passes the eggs out in faeces. To survive these eggs require warm moist conditions. When toilets are not used and random defaecation practised the humid tropics facilitate persistence of the disease.

The eggs penetrate the skin of people with bare feet, or of those who have other skin contacts with moist soil. The worm lodges in the large bowel and causes anaemia by drawing blood from its host. It obviously is a filth disease.

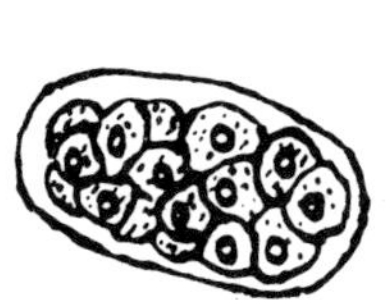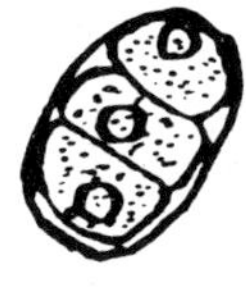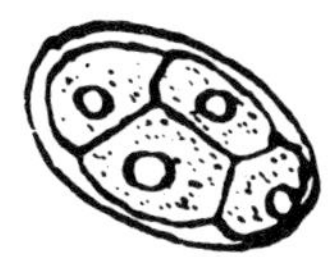

ENDNOTE 6

Dr R. Wood has gone a fair way towards sorting out the various microbes which probably caused the disease. The germs which caused the disease were apparently various. I doubt if we will ever know their exact nature. They caused acute painful infections of the eye, which sometimes temporarily blinded the victims. The great majority of patients recovered without any chronic ill effects.

However, a minority of patients with ophthalmia developed a painful condition which persisted. A few of these went blind. They suffered from true trachoma. Today in Australia the disease is confined to Aboriginal populations, but throughout the world it is still a major cause of blindness.[272]

ENDNOTE 7

When this Oration was given in 1969 I was justified in saying on p. 59 that public health was prevention practised by a community collectively. Now by modern Australian usage public health is deemed to be the study of health and disease in numbers of people and not in individuals.

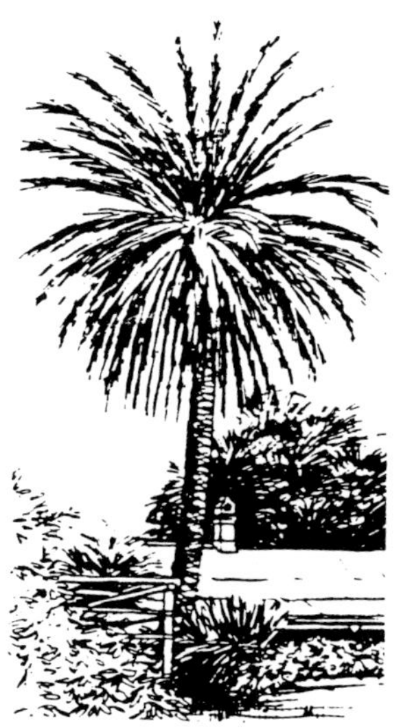

REFERENCES

1. **Trollope A.** *Australia*, **2nd Edit. Edwards PD and Joyce RB, Brisbane,** University of Queensland Press, 1967, pp 67, 87.

2. **Registrar-General.** Fifth Report: Registration of Births, Marriages and Deaths, 1865. *Votes and Proceedings of the Queensland Parliament 1865,* Brisbane, 1866.

3. **Haran J.** Appendix to Registrar-General's Report for 1865. *Votes and Proceedings of the Queensland Parliament 1865,* p 1286. Brisbane, 1866.

4. **Jee HC.** "A few remarks on Torres Strait", *Aust Med Gaz,* 1884, 3:223.

5. **Bolton GC.** *A Thousand Miles Away.* Australian National University and Jacaranda Press, Brisbane, 1963.

6. **Davidson BR.** *The Northern Myth,* 2nd Edit., Melbourne. Melbourne University Press, 1966.

7. **Cilento R and Lack C.** *Triumph in the Tropics,* Brisbane. Smith and Paterson, 1959, p 422.

8. **Lee DHK.** *Climate and Economic Development in the Tropics.* New York. Harper Bros, 1958, p 8.

9. **Huntington E.** *Civilization and Climate,* 3rd Edit., New Haven. Yale University Press, 1924.

10. **Brown NS.** *In* "The Development of Northern Australia". Report of a Symposium held at the University of New South Wales. Sydney. University of New South Wales, 1961.

11. **Harlin FW.** *Med J Aust,* 1915, 2:161.

12. **McCallum F.** Bionomics of Australian History. *Health,* 1926, 4.52.

13. **Editor.** *Aust Med Gaz,* 1896, 15: 73.

14. **Griffiths FG.** *Med J Aust,* 1915, 2: 241.

15. **Bolton GC.** *op. cit.* (p viii), p 21.

16. **Cilento R and Lack C.** *op. cit.* pp 422–423.

17. **Price G.** "White Settlers in the Tropics". New York. American Geographic Society, pp 16, 29, 148. 1939.

18. **Curtin PD.** "Epidemiology and the Slave Trade", *Political Science Quarterly,* LXXX, 1968, 3: 190–216.

19. **Price G.** *op. cit.* pp 4, 5, 227.

20. **Cilento R.** *The White Race in the Tropics.* Commonwealth Department of Health, Melbourne, 1925.

21. **Elkington JCS.** *Aust Med Gaz*, 1910, 29 : 614.
     Elkington JCS. "The Mesitzos of Kisar, Dutch East Indies,"1922, *Med J Aust* 1: 32.
     Elkington JCS. *Med J Aust* 1923, 2: 81.

22. **Rodenwaldt E.** *Med J Aust*, 1923, 2: 6.

23. **Encyclopaedia Britannica.** University of Chicago, 1964, 22: 497.

24. **Editor.** "The White Race in the Tropics", *Med J Aust,* 1945, 1: 85.

25. **Ewart K.** 1969. Personal communication, Department of Economics, University of Queensland.

26. **Hunt A.** Letter to Professor Harvey Sutton. *In* Records of Commonwealth Health Department, Canberra, 1933.

27. **Taylor G.** *The Control of Settlement by Humidity & Temperature,* Commonwealth Bureau of Meteorology, 1916.

28. **Taylor G.** *Australia,* 3rd Edit., London: Methuen & Co., 1945.
     Taylor G. Report of a Symposium on Man and Animals in the Tropics, held in Brisbane 1956. Canberra: Aust. Academy of Science, 1956.

29. **Price G.** *op. cit.,* 1939.

30. **Lee DHK.** Inaugural lecture. *Med J Aust,* 1936, 2: 707.
     Lee DHK. *A Basis for the Study of Man's Reaction to Tropical Climates.* Brisbane. University of Queensland Press, 1940.
     Lee DHK. *Physiological principles in Tropical Housing, with especial reference to Queensland.* Brisbane. University of Queensland Press, 1944.
     Lee DHK. *Human climatology and tropical settlement.* Brisbane. University of Queensland Press, 1947.

31. **Cilento RW.** *Med J Aust,* 1933, 1: 421.

32. **Macpherson RK.** *Tropical Fatigue.* Brisbane. University of Queensland Press, 1949.

33. **Queensland Government Gazette,** 24th February 1921.
     Queensland Government Gazette, 27th April, 1921.
     Queensland Government Gazette, 11th November, 1921.

34. **Bureau of Meteorological Services.** "Queensland Coastal Weather" and "Tropical Cyclones in the Queensland Region", cyclostyled. Brisbane. Queensland Regional Office, 1969.

35. **Bureau of Census and Statistics.** *Commonwealth Year Book 1966.* Commonwealth Government, Canberra, 1966.

36. **Lee DHK.** *op. cit.,* 1940, p 72.

37. **Lee DHK.** *op. cit.,* 1940.

38. **Stokes J.** *Discoveries in Australia; with an account of the Coasts and Rivers explored and surveyed during the Voyage of HMS Beagle in the years 1837–43.* London. T & W Boone, 1846.

39. **Votes and Proceedings of the Queensland Parliament 1868-69.** Brisbane, p 447.

40. **Bureau of Census and Statistics.** *Commonwealth Year Book 1958.* Commonwealth Government, Canberra, p 29.

41. **Lee DHK.** *op. cit.,* 1940, p 61.
    Lee DHK. Physiological Objectives in Hot Weather Housing. Washington, DC. USA. *Housing and Home Furnishing Agency,* 1953, p 69.

42. **Barrett J.** *Med J Aust.,* 1935, 1: 229.

43. **Brown NS.** *op. cit.,* p 105.

44. **Price G.** *op. cit.,* pp 73, 75.

45. **Bolton GC.** *op. cit.*

46. **CSIRO Div. Report 59/2** (cyclostyled). Canberra, 1959.

47. **Blainey G.** *Mines in the Spinifex.* Sydney. Angus & Robertson, 1960.

48. **Deputy Commonwealth Statistician.** *Queensland Year Book 1968.* Bureau of Census and Statistics, Brisbane, 1969.

49. **Bolton GC.** *op. cit.,* p 19.

50. **Phillips G.** *In Early Days in North Queensland,* (see next reference). Foreword, Sydney, 1903.

51. **Palmer E.** *Early Days in North Queensland.* Sydney. Angus & Robertson, 1903.

52. **Clarke PS.** Appendix E1 to Report of Commissioner of Public Health (Queensland) for the year ending 30th June 1913.

53. **Waterson DB.** *Squatter, Selector and Storekeeper.* Sydney. Sydney University Press, 1968, p 192.

54. **Votes and Proceedings of the Queensland Parliament 1879,** Vol 1.

55. **Aust Med Gaz.,** 1889–1890, 9 : 122, 259.

56. **Salter AE.** "Pearl Diving from a Physician's point of view". *Transactions of Intercolonial Medical Congress of Australasia*, Third Session, 1892, p 168.

57. **Chisholm A.** Editor, Roth, Walter Edmund, *Australian Encyclopaeida*, Sydney. Angus & Robertson, 1958, Vol. 7.

58. **Price G.** *op. cit.*, p 30.

59. **Haran J.** *Votes and Proceedings of Queensland Parliament 1867*, Vol. 1, p 1461.

60. **Anonymous.** *Med J Aust.*, 1919. 1: 477.

61. **Cilento R.** *Health*, 1926. January and March.

62. **Editor.** Health in Tropical Queensland, 1910, *Aust Med Gaz.*, 29: 614.

63. **Australian Hookworm Campaign 1919-1924.** Final Report (cyclostyled). Copy in Bancroft Library, University of Queensland, p 82.

64. **Commissioner of Public Health (Q).** Annual Reports for the years ending 30th June: 1904, p 10. 1908, p 29; 1912, p 12; and 1913.

65. **Cilento R.** The White Man in the Tropics. Melbourne. Commonwealth Department of Health, 1925, pp 35, 95.

66. **Commissioner of Public Health (Q).** Annual Report for the year ending 30th June 1913.

67. **Mitchell P.** A Short Medical History of Townsville. *Health*, 1925, March.

68. **Lambert SM.** *A Doctor in Paradise*, Dent & Son, Fourth Australian Edition, 1946, p 12.

69. **Borrie WD.** Italians and Germans in Australia; study in assimilation. Melbourne. Cheshire for ANU., 1954.

70. **Silverstone H, Campbell CB, Hosking CS, Lang LP, Richardson RG.** Regional Studies in Skin Cancer, North Western Queensland. First Report, *Med J Aust.*, 1963. 1: 312.
    Silverstone H and Gordon D. Regional Studies in Skin Cancer, Second Report: Wet Tropical and Sub-tropical Coasts of Queensland. *Med J Aust.*, 1966. 2: 733.

71. **Ferry TA.** *Ferry Report*. Report of Royal Commission to inquire into and report on the social and economic effects of the increase in numbers of aliens in North Queensland. *Votes and Proceedings of the Queensland Parliament 1925, 3: 25*.

72. **Hempel JA.** "Italians in Queensland", cyclostyled. Dept of Demography, Australian National University, Canberra, 1959.

73.   **Australian Hookworm Campaign 1919–1924.** Final Report, *ibid.*

74.   **Deputy–Commonwealth Statistician.** *Queensland Year Book 1968*, Brisbane. Bureau of Census and Statistics.

75.   **McGregor C.** *Profile of Australia.* Ringwood, Victoria. Penguin, 1968, p 357.

76.   **Breinl A.** Yearly report January-December 1919 of the Australian Institute of Tropical Medicine. Commonwealth of Australia, 1920, p 6.

77.   **Mitchell P.** *Health*, 1925, *ibid.*

78.   **Reports of the Registrar-General of Births, Marriages and Deaths** as appearing in *Votes and Proceedings of the Queensland Parliament for years 1866 to 1915.*

79.   **Registrar-General (Q).** *ibid,* Annual Report, *Votes and Proceedings 1876,* p 463.

80.   **Registrar-General.** *ibid,* Annual Report, *Votes and Proceedings 1878,* p 949.

81.   **Votes and Proceedings of the Queensland Parliament 1877,** Vol 2. 666-668.

82.   **Hunt JS.** Notes on the Demography of North Queensland. *Transactions of the Third Session of the Intercolonial Medical Congress, 1892,* p 594.

83.   **Editor.** Report of a delegation to Northcote, the Governor-General, while he was in North Queensland. *Aust Med Gaz.,* 1907. 26: 312.

84.   **Breinl A.** Annual Report of the AITM for the year 1910, p 15.

85.   **Breinl A.** *ibid.*

86.   **Breinl A.** The Stewart Lecture. *Med J Aust.,* 1915. 1: 547.

87.   **Breinl A.** *ibid,* 1920. See Reference 86.

88.   **Maplestone PA.** "Research in Australia", *Med J Aust.,* 1922. 1: 476, 527, 590, 682.

89.   **Mitchell P.** *ibid,* 1925.

90.   **Cilento R and Baldwin A.** Malaria in Australia. *Med J Aust.,* 1930. 1: 274.

91.   **Ford E.** The malaria problem in Australia and the Australian Pacific Territories. *Med J Aust.,* 1950, 1: 749.

92.   **Derrick EH.** The Challenge of North Queensland Fevers. *Aust Ann Med.,* 1957, 6: 173.

92a. **Lumley G and Taylor FH.** "Dengue", Sydney, Commonwealth of Australia. School of Public Health and Tropical Medicine, 1943.

92b. **White GV.** Ulcerating Granuloma of the Pudenda. *Proceedings of the Sixth Session of the Intercolonial Medical Congress of Australasia,* 1902, 183 (see also pp 178, 180, 185).

92c. **Nimmo JR.** The White Man in the Tropics. *Med J Aust.,* 1935. 1: 383.

93. **Cilento R and Lack C.** *ibid* p 423.

94. **Derrick EH.** *ibid,* 1957.

95. **James R.** "Remarks on the Fevers and Diseases of Tropical Queensland", *Aust Med Gaz.,* 1891. 10: 301.

96. **Dyson TS.** Malarial Fevers of Tropical Queensland. *Transactions of Intercolonial Med. Congress,* Second Session, 1889, p 64.

97. **White JA.** On the fevers of the Gulf of Carpentaria. *Aust Med J,* 1867. 12: 361.

98. **Cumpston JHL and McCallum F.** The history of intestinal infections (and typhus fever) in Australia, 1788-1923. Melbourne. Australian Dept of Health, H.J. Green, Government Printer, 1927.

99. **Cilento R and Baldwin A.** *op. cit.,* 1930.

100. **Nisbet ATH.** *Proceedings Australasian Med. Congress,* Ninth Session, 1911, p 533.
Nisbet ATH. *Transactions Aust. Med. Congress,* Eleventh Session, 1920, p 54.

101. **Hunt JS.** *ibid,* 1892.

102. **Bolton GC.** *ibid.*

103. **Hardie D.** Notes on some of the more common diseases in Queensland in relation to atmospheric conditions, 1887-1891. Brisbane, Government Printer, 1893.

104. **Derrick EH.** *ibid,* 1957.

105. **Palmer E.** *ibid,* 1957.

106. **Anonymous (Weitemeyer TPL).** "Missing Friends – 1871–1890", London T Fisher, Unwin, 1892, pp 156, 204, 220.

107. **Clarke PS.** *ibid.*

108. **Hardie D.** *ibid,* 1893.

109. **Hunt JS.** *ibid,* 1892.

110. **Brisbane Courier,** 1875. November 17.

111. **Brisbane Courier**, 1875. October 28.

112. **Brisbane Courier**, 1875. October 28; November 6, 17, 19, 20, 26, 27; December 11, 13, 17.

113. **Brisbane Courier**, 1875. December 13.

114. **Landsborough Papers.** Brisbane. Oxley Library.

115. **Anonymous (Weitemeyer TPL)** *ibid*, 1892.

116. **Keesing N.** Edit. *Gold Fever*. Sydney. Angus & Robertson, 1967.

117. **Derrick EH.** *ibid*, 1957.

118. **Mitchell P.** *ibid*, 1925.

119. **Elkington JSC.** "Quarantine in Queensland", *Aust Med Gaz.*, 1912, 31: 433.

120. **Brisbane Courier**, 1866. July 5, 11, 14; September 8; November 9, 10, 12, 13; December 19.

121. **Palmer E.** *ibid*, p 72.

122. **Commissioner of Public Health (Q).** Annual Report for the year ending 30th June 1910, p 6.

123. **Gordon D.** Ballow and the *Emigrant* Incident. *Med J Aust.*, 1966, 1:483.

124. **Editor.** Report on Wray's death. *Aust Med Gaz.*, 1902. 21: 280.

125. **Brisbane Courier**, 1902. May 4, p 4.

126. **Derrick EH.** *ibid*, 1957.

127. **Cotter TJP and Sawers WC.** A laboratory and epidemiological investigation of an outbreak of Weil's disease in Northern Queensland. *Med J Aust.*, 1934. 2 . 597.

128. **Morrissey GC.** The occurrence of leptospirosis (Weil's disease) in Australia. *Med J Aust.*, 1934, 2: 496.

129. **Johnson DW.** The Australian leptospiroses. *Med J Aust.*, 1950. 2: 724.

130. **Holthouse, Hector.** *River of Gold*, Sydney. Angus & Robertson, 1967.

131. **Votes and Proceedings of the Queensland Parliament.** 1876, 2: 407, 521; 1877, 2: 667, 757; 1878, 1: 947; 1879, 1: 26.

132. **Brisbane Courier**, 1877. May 16, June 27.

133. **Derrick EH.** *ibid*, 1957.

134. **Cumpston JHL and McCallum F.** *op. cit.* 1927, p 291.

135. **Bureau of Census and Statistics.** Deaths 1967. Commonwealth of Australia.

136. **Ford E.** *ibid,* 1950.

137. **Black RH.** Deaths from malaria on the Australian mainland. *Med J Aust.,* 1955. 1: 387.

138. **Derrick EH.** *ibid,* 1957.

139. **Landsborough Papers,** No 6 Field Book. Brisbane. Oxley Library.

140. **Gunther J.** The Thomson Lecture for 1969. University of Queensland, unpublished, 1969.

141. **Cilento R and Baldwin A.** *ibid,* 1930.

142. **President.** *Aust Med Gaz.,* 1893, 12: 50.

143. **O'Brien RA.** Anaemia in Ancyclostomiasis and Malaria. *Transactions of the Eighth Session of the Aust Med Congress, 1908,* Vol 1, p 241; and Ancyclostomiasis and other tropical diseases in Queensland, *ibid,* 2: 324, 326.

144. **Commissioner of Public Health (Q).** Annual Reports for years ending 30th June, 1904, p 5; 1909, p 3; 1910, p 5.
Editor, Tropical Diseases in Australia. *Aust Med Gaz.,* 1913, 34: 556.

145. **Final Report of the Australian Hookworm Campaign 1919-1924.** *ibid.*

146. **Waite JH and Neilson IL.** A study of the effects of hookworm infection upon the mental development of North Queensland school children. *Med J Aust.,* 1919, 1: 1.

147. **Commissioner of Public Health (Q).** Annual Report for the year ending 30th June 1911, p 7.

148. **Final Report of the Australian Hookworm Campaign 1919-1924.** *ibid.*

149. **Sawyer WA.** Hookworm in Australia. *Med J Aust.,* 1921. 1: 148.

150. **Hogg JB.** A case of death from Anaemia due to Ankylostoma Duodenale. *Aust Med Gaz,* 1889, 8: 133.

151. **Derrick EH.** *ibid,* 1957.

152. **Director-General of Health and Medical Services (Q).** Annual Report 1968-69, p 19.

153. **Gordon D.** Sickness and Death at the Moreton Bay Convict Settlement. *Med J Aust.,* 1963. 2: 473.

154. **May JM.** *The Ecology of the Human Disease.* New York. M.D. Publications, 1958, pp 276, 297, 298.

155. **Hunt JS**. *ibid*, 1892.

156. **Editor**. Health in Tropical Queensland. *Aust Med Gaz.*, 1910. 29: 614.

156a. **Carmichael GC and Silverstone H**. "The Epidemiology of Skin Cancer in Queensland: the incidence". *Brit J Cancer*, 1961. 15: 409-424.

156b. **Silverstone H** *et al. ibid*, 1963.

156c. **Silverstone H and Gordon D**. 1966.

157. **Hunt JS**. *ibid*, 1892.

158. **Lee DHK**. Human Climatology and Tropical Settlement. Brisbane. University of Queensland, 1947, p 20.

159. **Silverstone H** *et al, ibid*, 1963.

160. **Silverstone H and Gordon D**. *ibid*, 1966.

161. **Brisbane Courier**. 1877, December 15.

162. **Brisbane Courier**. 1878, May 30.

163. **Brisbane Courier**. 1875, November 17.

164. **Cumpston JH and McCallum F**. "History of Plague in Australia 1900-1925". Commonwealth Dept of Health, 1926, p 29.

165. **Breinl A**. *Transactions of the Ninth Session of the Australasian Medical Congress*, 1911, p 529.

166. **Jackson ES**. Notes on Filaria in Queensland. *Aust Med Gaz.*, 1910. 29: 231.

167. **Commissioner of Public Health (Q)**. Annual Report for the year ending 30th June 1909. App. C, p 16.

168. **Thompson JA**. "Contributions to the History of Leprosy in Australia". London. MacMillan & Co., 1897.

169. **Cook C**. "The Epidemiology of Leprosy in Australia". Commonwealth Dept of Health, 1927.

170. **Nisbet ATH**. *ibid*, 1911.

171. **Breinl A**. *Aust Med Gaz.*, 1913. 34: 556.

172. **Osborne W**. *Aust Med Gaz.*, 1912. 31.540.

173. **Osborne W**. *Med J Aust.*, 1916. 2: 413.

174. **Osborne W**. *Transactions of Aust Med Congress*, Eleventh Session, 1920. 2: 87.

175. **Editor**. *Aust Med Gaz.*, 1911. 30: 519.

176. **Hunt A.** *ibid*, 1933.

177. **Breinl A.** *Transactions of Aust Med Congress*, Eleventh Session, 1920. pp 49, 558.

178. **Breinl A and Young WJ.** Tropical Australia and its Settlement. *Med J Aust.*, 1919, 1: 353, 375, 395.

179. **Nisbet ATH.** *ibid*, 1920.

180. **Macpherson RK.** *ibid*, p 143.

181. **Elliot C.** *Transactions of Aust Med Congress*, Eleventh Session, 1920. 2: 317.

182. **Maplestone PA.** *ibid*, 1922.

183. **Editor.** *Med J Aust.*, 1920. 2: 291.

184. **Macfarlane WV.** Water and Salt turnover in cane cutters working on the coastal sub-tropics of Australia. *Med J Aust.*, 1957, 2: 229.

185. **Burry AF.** A profile of renal disease in Queensland; results of an autopsy survey. *Med J Aust.*, 1966. 1: 826.

186. **Patrick RP.** Heights and Weights of Queensland school children with special reference to the tropics: a report of an anthropometric survey by Queensland school health services. *Med J Aust.*, 1951, 2: 324.

187. **Huntington E.** *Mainsprings of Civilization.* New York. John Wiley & Sons, 1945, p 192.

188. **Goldsmith F.** "The necessity for the Study of Tropical Medicine in Australia". *Transactions of the Sixth Session of the Intercolonial Med. Congress of Australasia, 1902.* p 178; and *Aust Med Gaz.*, 21: 131.

189. **Transactions of the Eleventh Session of Aust Med. Congress,** Brisbane, 1920. 2: 39, 317, 558, 559, 568.

190. **Transactions of the Eighth Session of the Aust Med. Congress,** Melbourne, 1908. 100-103; *Aust Med Gaz.*, 1912, 31: 161; Commissioner of Public Health (Q). Annual Report for year ending 30th June 1909, p 2; *Aust Med Gaz.*, 1907, 26: 312.

191. **Breinl A.** *Med J Aust.*, 1919. 1: 353, 375, 395.

192. **Report of the Commissioner of Public Health (Q) for the year ending 30th June 1908.**

193. **Votes and Proceedings of the Queensland Parliament 1907.** 2. 53. Report on Plague.

194. **Commissioner of Public Health (Q).** Annual Reports for years ending 30th June 1901 to 1908. Also Annual Report for year ending 30th June 1917.

195. **Brisbane Courier.** 1901: April 17, 27; June 9; September 14, 18; 1902: March 15, 19, 21; April 1, 3, 4, 5, 7, 21; May 13, 16, 21, 28, 30; June 6, 13, 17, 18, 24. July 4, 12, 16; August 9, 16, 22; September 13, 24.

196. **Votes and Proceedings of the Queensland Parliament 1907.** *ibid.*

197. **Our correspondent, "Queensland".** *Aust Med Gaz.,* 1908, 22: 227.

198. **Brisbane Courier,** 1901. February 6.

199. **Commissioner of Public Health (Q).** Report submitted in July 1901. (This was for a half year only since the first Commissioner did not take up office until January 1901.)

200. **Commissioner of Public Health (Q).** Annual Reports for the years ending 30th June: 1911, p 7; 1912, p 8; 1914; 1915.

201. **Editor.** *Aust Med Gaz.,* 1913. 33: 227.

202. **Commissioner of Public Health (Q).** Annual Report for year ending 30th June 1916, p 10.

203. **Editor.** Tempting Providence. *Med J Aust.,* 1916. 1: 417.

204. **Hardie D.** *op. cit.*

205. **Editor.** Medical Appointments. *Aust Med Gaz.,* 1913. 34: 281.

206. **Waite JH.** *Med J Aust.,* 1918. 2: 505.

207. **Waite JH and Lambert SR.** Report of the AITM from 1st July to 31st December 1918.

208. **Lambert SR.** *op. cit.*

209. **Holmes MJ.** Hookworm Control in Australia. *Health,* 1925. 3: 45.

210. **Bearup AJ.** The Intensity and type of Hookworm Infestation in the Ingham District of North Queensland. *Med J Aust.,* 1931. 2: 65.

211. **Final Report of the Australian Hookworm Campaign.** *op. cit.*

212. **Lumley GF.** District serological groups of leptospirae causing leptospirosis as it occurs in Northern Queensland. *Med J Aust.,* 1937. 1: 654.

213. **Smith DJW.** Leptospirosis in Queensland. *Queensland Health,* 1964. I, No 5, p 1.

214. **Patrick RP.** Personal communication.

215. **Kennedy JM, Lulham CR and Gordon D.** Occupational fevers, Queensland, 1950-51. *Med J Aust,* 1952. 1: 360.

216. **Doherty R.** Annual Report of the Council of the Queensland Institute of Medical Research for the year ending 30th June 1955. Brisbane. State Health Department, 1955.

217. **Abrahams EW. and Silverstone H.** Epidemiological evidence of the presence of non-tuberculosis sensitivity to tuberculin in Queensland. *Tubercle*, 1961. 42: 487.

218. **Walker AS.** Edit. *Australia in the War of 1939-45*, Series V, Medicine. Vol. 1. Clinical problems of war, p 104. Canberra. Australian War Memorial, 1952.

219. **McLeod NJ.** *Transactions of the Eleventh Session Aust Med Congress*, 1920, p 330.

220. **Osborne WA.** *Transactions of the Eleventh Session Aust Med Congress*, 1920, p 97.

221. **Elkington JCS.** Report of the Commissioner of Public Health (Q), for year ending 30th June 1913.

222. **President.** First Presidential Address to North Queensland Medical Society. *Aust Med Gaz.*, 1889-90. 9 : 292.

223. **Editor.** *Med J Aust.*, 1915. 1 : 237, 252.

224. **Hunt A.** *ibid.*, 1933.

225. **Editor.** *Aust Med Gaz.*, 1907. 26: 240, 312.

226. **Editor.** *Aust Med Gaz.*, 1908. 27: 677.

227. **Editor et al.** Obituary TA Stuart, 1920. *Med J Aust.*, 1 . 215, 244, 247, 248, 249, 307, 326, 388, 474, 520, 559.

228. **Breinl A.** Report for the year 1911, AITM Sydney. Angus & Robertson, 1913.

229. **Editor.** *Aust Med Gaz.*, 1913. 34 : 15, 124.

230. **Editor et al.** Obituary TA Stuart, *ibid*, 1920.

231. **Editor.** *Med J Aust.*, 1920, 1: 493.

232. **Editor.** *Med J Aust.*, 1920. 2: 292.

233. **Breinl J.** Family papers, Townsville, 1969.

234. **Maplestone PA.** *op. cit.*, 1922.

235. **Editor.** *Med J Aust.*, 1922. 1 : 17.

236. **Editor.** *Med J Aust.*, 1922. 2: 739.

237. **Editor.** *Med J Aust.*, 1923. 1 : 17.

238. **Robin PD.** The British Medical Association in Queensland — origins and development (to 1945). Honours thesis, Dept of History, University of Queensland, 1966, p 156.

239. **Daily Mail**, 1933. July 25.

240. **Brisbane Courier,** 1933. July 25.

241. **Courier Mail,** 1933. September 15, 19.

242. **Brisbane Telegraph,** 1933. September 16.

243. **Editor.** Report of the Royal Commission on Health. *Med J Aust.,* 1926. 1: 55.

244. **Maplestone PA.** *ibid,* 1922.

245. **Editor.** *Med J Aust.,* 1915. 1: 237, 252.

246. **Hunt A.** *ibid,* 1933.

247. **Registrar, University of Melbourne.** Personal communication, 24th June 1969.

248. **Registrar, University of Adelaide.** Personal communication, 9th June 1969.

249. **Archivist, University of Sydney.** Personal communication, 11th June 1969.

250. **Baldwin AH.** First course for the Australian Diploma in Tropical Medicine & Hygiene. *Health*, 1926. 4: 165.

251. **Purdy JS.** *Med J Aust.,* 1922. 1: 55.

252. **Macpherson RK.** *ibid.*

253. **Breinl A.** Report for year 1911 of AITM. *op. cit.*

254. **Derrick EH.** *ibid,* 1957.

255. **Editor.** *Aust Med Gaz.,* 1913. 34: 10, 423.

256. **Editor.** *Aust Med Gaz.,* 1912. 32: 23.

257. **Breinl A.** Report on Health and Disease in the Northern Territory 1912. Bull. No 1, March. Commonwealth Dept of External Affairs.

258. **Editor.** *Med J Aust.,* 1914. 2 : 85.

259. **Editor.** *Med J Aust.,* 1920. 1: 493.

260. **Editor.** *Med J Aust.,* 1920. 2 . 292.

261. **Anonymous.** Obituary Anton Breinl. *Aust J of Sci.,* 1944, August, p 28.

262. **Breinl J.** Personal communication, 1969.

263. **Editor.** *Aust Med Gaz.,* 1909. 28: 630.

264. **Dale HM.** *Fifty Years of Medicine: Advances in Therapeutics.* London. British Medical Association, 1950, p 44.

265. **Hunt A.** *ibid,* 1933.

266. **Anonymous.** Obituary A. Breinl, *Med J Aust.,* 1944. 2: 443.

266a. **Douglas RA.** Dr Anton Breinl and the Australian Institute of Tropical Medicine. *Med J Aust.,* 1977, I, 713-716; 748-751; 784-790.

267. **Standfast H.** Personal communication, 1969.

268. **Hardie D.** *ibid,* p 104.

269. **Price G.** *ibid,* p 68.

270. **Pearn J.** *In the Capacity of a Surgeon*, p 29, Dept of Child Health, Royal Children's Hospital, Herston, Brisbane, 1988.

271. **Doherty R.** Personal communication. 1979.

272. **Wood R.** p 245 in Pearn J and O'Carrigan C.(Edits.) *Australia's Quest for Colonial Health,* Royal Children's Hospital, Brisbane, 1983.

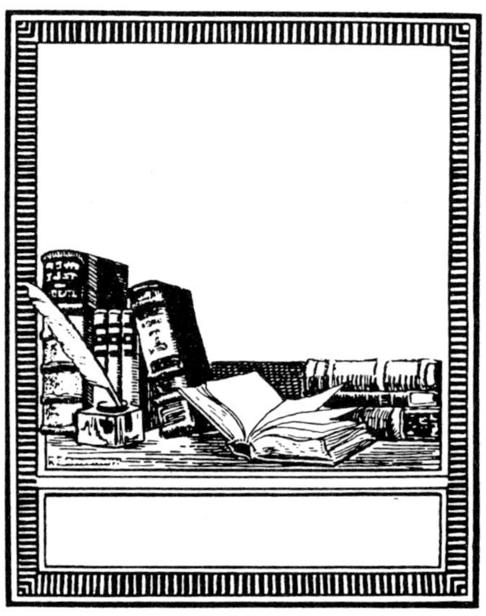

INDEX